Beating Food Allergies

Reversing Food Allergies with Vitamin and Nutrition Therapy

By

Dr. Dannielle P. MacDuff, ND

Acknowledgments

I wish to thank the many people who made this work possible;

- Dr. Bryan Cecil for you encouragement and support.

- My children; Sebastian, Clarissa and Brenna who constantly remind me how important it is to leave this place better than we found it.

- The entire team at DC Chiropractic and Wellness Center, without whose help much of the data in this work would not have been possible.

- Coach for inspiration and motivation that was given effortlessly, most likely without even knowing you were doing it.

Table of Contents

Introduction

We have been told that allergies cannot be cured, they are just something that we have to learn to live with if we are unfortunate enough to develop them. We are taught that avoidance is the only option for the treatment of food allergies. This book debunks those medical myths. In these pages we will explore the causes of food allergies and their associated diseases. We will also reveal how those allergies can be reversed, eliminated, and – dare I say- cured with simple food.

I first began this work as my doctoral thesis in naturopathic school. The subject matter is one that resonates with me because of my own allergies. In my twenties I developed a severe allergy to tree nuts. After enjoying my grandmother's pecan pie and nut encrusted cheese logs as well as snacking on pistachios as a staple in my diet for my entire life up to that point, I found myself in the emergency room after having Chinese food with friends one night. The dish contained walnuts which triggered an anaphylactic reaction. The reaction necessitated a trip to the hospital and a diagnosis of severe allergy to tree nuts.

For years after that incident I carried an Epipen for those occasions when accidental exposure occurred. Those of you familiar with these types of reaction, you already know that avoidance requires constant vigilance and ongoing education of those around you, particularly the staff at restaurants and other social events. I found myself frequently explaining that I have this severe allergy and that any cross contamination of my food had the potential of causing me to come down with a sudden case of death.

Exposure meant either stabbing myself or being stabbed by someone else with a 2 ½ inch needle attached to the Epipen which would deliver a dose of synthetic epinephrine into the blood stream to combat constriction of the airways that, if left unchecked, would result in suffocation. This was followed by a trip to the hospital where a "precautionary" dose of epinephrine was administered and I was kept for "observation".

The part of this experience that was most frustrating to me were the other effects of the epinephrine. It caused tachycardia – racing heartbeat, migraines and nausea, all of which lasted more than a day. Invariably, an 'attack' meant loss of work time, disruption of family and social life or any combination of the above. I was also disturbed to learn that an overdose of epinephrine can increase the rate of heart contractions to the point that the cardiac muscles tear, essentially causing the heart to explode. Not once had I ever been asked by emergency responders or hospital staff if I had administered my Epipen or what the dosage of that pen was. Eventually, I stopped going to the hospital, but rather administered the Epipen and stayed home where I could rest and monitor myself.

Several years ago, through a classmate in a Herbology class, I discovered an herb that could be used to combat anaphylaxis called Osha root. After some research of my own, I purchased the herb and proceeded to brew my first batch of Osha root *tincture*. I carried the tincture in

7

conjunction with my Epipen with me everywhere that I went. When I was exposed to nuts, I first took the tincture under my tongue and waited. If I needed it I could always use the Epipen as a backup. I never needed it. Within seconds of administering the tincture, I felt my airways open up and my breathing began to become less difficult. Within 20 minutes, I was back to normal and able to continue with whatever I had been doing prior to the attack. In addition, I did not experience any rapid heartbeat, nausea or migraines from using the herb and there was no risk of epinephrine overdose. I have not carried an Epipen for nearly 3 years as of the writing of this book.

That got me thinking. If chronic degenerative diseases can be reversed by rebalancing a person's nutrient levels, why could we not do the same with allergies? We can mitigate anaphylaxis with Osha Root – an herb, which is a food. It just made sense that we could correct the causes of allergies with food as well. This became the hypothesis for my dissertation as well as the clinical study conducted to as part of that same paper.

The decision to publish resulted from a memory of my grandmother telling me that we should leave this place better than we found it. After all, what good is knowledge if it is not shared? I believe that truth shared becomes wisdom and, that applied wisdom leads to an improved quality of life. So it seemed that it would be selfish not to record and publish what I had learned.

The information in this book is not meant to diagnosis any condition or as a plan for the treatment of any condition, nor is it a substitute for the advice of a trained professional. Rather, the contents of this book are meant to provide you with knowledge so that you are better equipped to make informed decisions and be an active participant in your own health care. This book is also meant to offer hope to those who suffer from these allergies and other conditions, to show you that there are more options available than the ones offered by our western medical system

At Phoenix House Wellness Center, through our Breed Hope Campaign, we strive to bring knowledge of the viable, effective natural options in health care that are available and to offer healing and hope to those who have been told by allopathic(medical) doctors that 'there is nothing [more] to be done.' That 'you are just going to have to live with it.' In many cases these same people are told that the condition will probably get worse. I am here to tell you that that does not have to be the case. There are other health care choices and there is hope.

This book is the first of many tools design to do that very thing…Breed Hope!

Happy Healing,

Dr. Danni

Chapter 1

A Look at Allergies

What is an allergic reaction?

An allergic reaction is a normal immune response. The body senses an invader-anything that presents a threat to the body, and an immune response is then triggered that response will destroy, isolate or rapidly expel the invader from the body, provided out immune system in functioning well. Many of these responses are touted as malfunction of the body and we spend billions of dollars each year trying to suppress these 'symptoms'. In the case of food allergies the body lacks the tools to process the food and damaged or defective enzymes send erroneous signals to the body that an invader is present which, begins the process of protecting us from harm.

Signs of an immune response.

The normal immune functions; fever, cough, mucus, vomiting and diarrhea, swelling and sneezing have been mislabeled as dysfunction of the body. We are inundated everyday with marketing that tells us to purchase products that will suppress [relieve] these symptoms. Unfortunately, suppressing these symptoms interrupts the immune process and stops the elimination of the antagonistic substance which then remains in the body and usually comes back stronger, producing symptoms that are stronger. We then repeat the cycle of suppressing the symptoms without addressing the cause of the symptoms.

Fever

Fever is probably the most important immune response of the body and it is the one that is most suppressed. Fever is the body's destruction method for bacteria, virus and most foreign invaders. Yet we are taught to reduce a fever and seek medical assistance to reduce body temperatures of more than 103°F. This practice prohibits the body from ever reaching optimal temperature for the eradication of these invaders.

Think of your body as a Pac Man board. The ghosts represent the bacteria, virus, or other invader attacking the body. Pac Man represents your immune cells. Under normal conditions, if Pac Man runs into the ghosts, he dies. The immune cell is not strong enough to fight off the invaders. Under these conditions, we would easily become overwhelmed by harmful microbes, the body would succumb to the damage these organisms do and we would soon die. But Not To Worry! Our bodies have a natural boost to our immune function. I call it the Power Pellet Zone.

When Pac Man Eats the Power Pellet, two things happen. First, Pac Man becomes super charged, increasing in speed and strength. Simultaneously, the ghosts slow down and begin to blink-they get weaker. In the body our immune cells speed up and start to 'hunt' the invaders, reaching out with tentacles that engulf the invaders & draw them into the 'mouth' of the immune cell where the microbe is digested

11

and delivered to the waste system of the body for elimination. The invaders also slow down, can't reproduce and many die off on their own because the rise in body temperature has become inhospitable to the metabolic systems of these invaders.

Where is the Power Pellet Zone, you ask? Between 103°F and 104°F. The best thing to do with a fever is to stay hydrated, bundle up and sweat it out. Applying a cool cloth to the base of the skull on young children will eliminate the concern of overheating the brain stem and causing brain damage.

Mucus and Congestion

Mucus and congestion are described as an inconvenience and nuisance and suppressed almost as readily as a fever. There are dozens of decongestant products on drug store shelves designed to stop the production of congestion causing mucus.

The body produces mucus all the time. It is necessary for protecting smooth tissues in the digestive tract, nasal cavities and other orifices. Its purpose is to create a protective barrier that prohibits harmful substances from being absorbed through the delicate membranes in these areas and causing damage. The production of excess mucus is an indication something is antagonizing those tissues. The mucus encapsulates the invader and removes it from the body via a runny nose, or loose, mucus laden stool. Congestion occurs when we are not adequately hydrated and the mucus becomes thick, sticky and unable to be easily excreted from the body. Consuming enough water to maintain proper hydration ensures that the mucus is the appropriate consistency to be eliminated from the body.

Coughs and Sneezing

Coughs and sneezing are a clear sign that the body is being attacked, particularly in the respiratory system. Both a cough and a sneeze are the body's way of rapidly expelling harmful substances from the body. A signal is sent to the immune system that there is something very dangerous in the body and we need to get rid of it fast. The threat is then isolated by engulfing it in mucus and, then putting it on the rocket train out of the body via a cough, when the invader is in the lung or lower airways. A sneeze is produced to expel invaders in the upper airways.

Vomiting and Diarrhea

I think the two most miserable immune responses are vomiting and diarrhea. Both are the violent evacuation of toxic substances from the digestive tract of the body. The digestive system begins to breakdown what we have consumed and suddenly recognizes some sort of poison in the body. A red alert is sounded and the body initiates reflexes that eliminate the toxins in one of two ways. For toxins still in the stomach, it's coming back up and vomiting occurs. If the toxicity has made its way to the intestines, a rapid evacuation of the bowel with occur. Additional water is rushed into the stool to make sure all of the toxins are flushed from the body and nothing is left behind in the gut tissue where it will be reabsorbed and cause more damage.

Swelling

There is one more immune response that can be life threatening and on those occasions, requires extra attention to avoid death. Swelling. When we are attacked by some environmental antagonist such as insect stings or chemicals, the body converts the amino acid histidine into histamine. The histamine is then sent to the affected area with lymph fluid to encapsulate the toxin and isolate it while the white blood cells mount an attack. Typically this results in localized swelling and is not life threatening. Sometime, as in the case of severe allergic reaction which creates an anaphylactic response, the signal is sent to close off all possible point of entry to the body. When this happens, swelling of the airways occurs restricting respiration and can lead to asphyxiation or suffocation.

Types of Allergies

While allergies may manifest as a wide variety of symptoms, they are typically classified into two categories; minor food intolerances and anaphylactic or deadly allergies.

Food Intolerances

Food intolerances may manifest such symptoms as indigestion, fatigue, minor skin eruptions and bloating, food coma, feeling of heaviness in the chest, excessive phlegm, congestion, inflamed tonsils, colic, mental and emotional distress, hiatal hernia, addiction, headaches, hair loss, nausea, vomiting, vision impairment, bone pain, psoriasis, liver enlargement, skin problems, mood changes, trouble concentrating, trouble regulating blood sugar, neuropathy, adrenal exhaustion, asthma, depression, anemia, kidney stones, cystitis, loss of muscular control, migraines, senility, MS and Parkinson's like symptoms, trouble regulating blood pressure, chronic pulmonary infections, impaired memory function, muscle spasms, angina and clotting malfunction, just to name a few.

These symptoms often result in a misdiagnosis as food allergies are not accepted in the medical community as a cause of metabolic dysfunction, and because the allopathic community does not have a treatment protocol for food allergies. Doctors are limited to treating severe reactions for food allergies. The concept of correcting the cause of these allergies is foreign to the majority of medical doctors. As a result, the variety of symptoms created by food intolerances often are grouped together to render an entirely different diagnosis for which the treatment is ineffective, or the symptoms are addressed individually. Again, this results in an ineffective treatment because the treatment is based on symptomology and not on cause. Food Intolerances, left unchecked, can escalate into more serious diseases. The recent increase of gut disorder diagnosis is a prime example of the escalation of intolerances into severe conditions. Often, Celiac disease can be traced back to many years of early signs of wheat intolerance symptoms that were either misdiagnosed or completely dismissed. Over time, the ongoing exposure to the allergen produces more severe symptoms until it is eventually debilitating. The patient is then diagnosed with Celiac's Disease. In truth, these types of diseases are not actually diseases, but very severe allergic responses.

I recently had a perfect example of this in my clinic. A woman came to see me who seemed to be suffering from every possible malady in the books. She had been diagnosed with possible rheumatoid arthritis, chronic fatigue, suspected fibromyalgia, gastrointestinal issues and various other intermittent chronic conditions. The ongoing pain in her body was beginning to affect her emotionally and mentally. She struggled to deal with the smallest of stresses and she was beginning to exhibit signs of depression. She was also extremely frustrated with the lack of result that she was getting from multiple doctors who could not give her an explanation that made sense, nor did any of the medication provide relief or improvement to her condition.

She had begun to change the way that she ate. Consuming a diet of more whole foods and far less processed packaged foods. This is when I met her. In my office, I offer 10 minute 'can you help me?' consultations at no charge. A member of the clinics team had convinced her to come to the office for one of these consults.

During that 10 minute consult she told me her story, in near tears. I asked her what she wanted to gain from working with me. Her response was desperate; "I want my life back. I can't do anything anymore!" I explained to here that I could help and that the next step would be to bring her in for a full exam. At that exam I would check for food allergies, determine nutrient levels, and examine her nails tongue and eyes for signs of digestive stress, malnutrition, poor absorption, inflammation, toxicity and low organ function. I also explained that at that first visit we would be determining the underlying cause of all of her symptoms so that we could develop a plan to correct the cause and there by eliminate the symptoms. She scheduled for the exam and returned a few days later for her appointment, husband in tow.

After we had finished the exam, it was determined that, in addition to being chronically dehydrated, she also suffered from multiple food allergies, ongoing gut toxicity, poor absorption and her internal pH was too far to the acidic side of the scale. All of which contributed to her on going symptoms and had led to a vicious cycle of chronic toxicity and nutritional deficiency- the cause!

Before the end of that first visit we discussed changes that needed to be made in order to give the body time to rest and reset. We set a daily water consumption goal to correct the dehydration, implemented several herbal teas and infused waters to balance the internal pH and provide much needed nutrients to the body while gently beginning to flush out and eliminate toxins from the body's tissues. I instructed her to eliminate allergen foods completely from her diet and she was given instructions on proper food combination to ensure optimal digestion and utilization of nutrients so that nutritional deficiencies could be corrected. Finally a follow up visit was scheduled for three weeks later.

When I walked into the room for that follow up visit, the changes in this woman were immediately evident. She was smiling, her skin looked better and there was a healthier glow to her. She began to tell me about her progress. Her sleep had improved, she had much less pain, bloating and feelings of just being 'off'. Her husband commented "this is the first time in years that I have been able to walk into the room and not find her in tears from the pain. She even offered to help carry a large pantry cabinet into the house. Three months ago that never would have happened, I wouldn't even think of asking. But she offered and we did it"

This couple then thanked me and told me that I had been the first doctor to show an interest in finding the cause of her troubles and offer a solution. All of the others had only offered pharmaceuticals as a solution. Medications which she stated had no effect on anything that she was experiencing, but did cause other symptoms.

Sadly this scenario is not a rare occurrence in my office. Most of my patients come to me frustrated and feeling very hopeless about the possibility of healing. Many remain misdiagnosed or undiagnosed and continue to suffer

Anaphylactic Allergies

Anaphylactic allergies on the other hand are often life threatening with symptoms that include swelling of tissues which may constrict or completely block airways and, if not attended to immediately, can lead to asphyxiation and death. It is believed that this type of allergy is caused by amino acid deficiency and a miscommunication in the nervous system of enzymatic directive.

This type of allergy, like many other metabolic dysfunction, often develops after a viral infection that has disrupted production of healthy enzymes and appropriate conversion of the amino acid histidine to histamine. Another theory is that the anaphylactic reaction is the end stage reaction of an intolerance that has not been corrected and became chronic producing more severe reactions with each exposure to the allergen. This reaction is a signal from the body to take note and take action. It is a very effective signal, I believe, as the threat of death tends to get our attention.

Food allergies are caused by nutritional deficiency. Wheat in particular may be caused by a deficiency of EFA's, Vitamin F, Magnesium and the amino acid histidine. Histidine is important in immune function as it is converted to histamine during an allergic reaction.

Many Do Not Know That They Have Food Allergies

It has been my clinical experience that a large percentage of people are unknowingly suffering from food allergies. Over the past three years working with hundreds patients, nearly all had food intolerances. Some individuals tested positive to nearly all of the 12 groups for which he/she was tested. Among patients seen at my clinic, wheat, corn, dairy and citrus groups where the most common allergies for which patients tested positive. Many with wheat allergies also had allergies to rice, corn and yeast groups. As you can see from

19

Table 1-1, this can limit food choices when selecting from those choices most prevalent in the Standard American Diet. Many with wheat allergies also indicate suffering from one or more of the following; seasonal allergies, chemical sensitivities, sensitivities to animal dander and asthma.

Wheat is not only in breads and other baked goods, but is used as filler in many packaged and processed foods. Foods such as sausages, bologna and luncheon meats as well as meatloaf, meat patties and breaded meats may contain wheat as a filler ingredient. Maltose, modified food starch, hydrolyzed protein and maltodextrin are all corn derivatives. Soy is another such filler. It is listed as one of the top 7 allergy foods and is also the most widely use filler in products like protein bars and gluten free products. According to Ingrid Malmheden 'children with severe allergies to peanuts should avoid intake of soy protein.'[1]

Those seen at my clinic complain of a wide range of symptoms including those of chronic arthritis, digestive trouble, chronic fatigue, seasonal allergies, migraines, sluggishness, mental fatigue, general fogginess and almost always have secondary conditions that are both caused by food allergies and exacerbated by them.

Table 1-1[*2]

Food Allergy by Group	Vitamin Antidote	Mineral Antidote	Amino Acid Antidote
Yeast Series: yeast, barley, cherry, millet, potatoes, prunes, raisins, rye and walnuts	B7, B6	Zinc	Lysine
Rice Series: all rice, cinnamon, curry, blueberry, grapes, strawberries, watermelon, wine, and pumpkin	B6, B12	Manganese	Arginine, proline
Wheat, feathers, wool, dust, detergents, cat and dog dander	EFA's, F-linoleic	Magnesium	Histidine
Corn	EFA's	Magnesium, Potassium	Histidine
Fat Series: meat fats, vegetables, cosmetics	Biotin	Sulfur	Methionine, cysteine, taurine, glutathione, threonine, carnitine
Oatmeal Series: oatmeal, sesame	Folic acid, B12	Iron	Ciruilline
Milk	D	Potassium	Aspartic acid, asparagine
Citrus Series: oranges, lemons, limes, grapefruit, tomatoes, pineapple,	B5	Calcium	Serine

tangerines, and cantaloupe			
Peppers, peaches, pears, plumes, nectarines	Niacin	Phosphorus	L'Glutamine
Nightshades: tobacco, potatoes, eggplant, peppers, tomatoes	Niacin	Sulfur	
Lettuce	Sodium deficiency indicator for asthmatics		
Fish oil	Used as a source of vitamins A & D in supplements. Tested to determine if this supplement is acceptable for individual.		

The Growing Number of Young Children Diagnosed With Serious Food Allergies

Prior to 1993 the instances of food allergies in young people under the age of 18 was dramatically lower than those in the same age group being diagnosed currently. Currently, it is estimated that 1 in 13 children suffer from severe food allergies. One study from the CDC states that 'food allergies among children increased approximately 50% between 1997 and 2011'.[3] According to the European Academy of Allergy and Clinical Immunology (EAACI), the number of children admitted to hospitals in Europe for severe allergic reaction to foods has risen seven-fold over the past decade.[4]

Studies show the number of children living with peanut allergy appears to have tripled between 1997 and 2008.[5] In another study released in 2008, reported food allergies increased 18% among children under the age of 18 between 1997 and 2007.[6] While this increase in diagnosed food, severe allergies among children continues to increase each year, there seems to be no explanation for the increase. Doctors do not offer correction of the allergy; instead, the patient is usually advised that an avoidance approach to managing the condition be implemented. It is the author's belief that this trend should not continue.

I believe this practice to be a disservice to both the children with the allergy and the parents of those children. With the knowledge that we currently have about reversing metabolic dysfunction, there is no excuse for not offering vitamin and nutrition therapy as a solution. So, why is it not? Currently, American Scientific method views recovery from disease using natural medicine, particularly vitamin and nutrition therapy as *anecdotal evidence* at best and *placebo effect* at worst. In the spirit of healing, I would like to defer to what is called evidence based medicine.

Evidence Based Medicine can be interpreted in several ways. Allopathic medicine considers this by be any medical procedure or finding that can be tested in a laboratory and have the results repeated in that setting. I would like offer a natural alternative to this definition. If a treatment is administered to a patient, and the patient improves or recovers, then there is evidence that the therapy is effective. What remains a point of contention among the scientific community, is that this definition cannot be broadly applied to groups of individuals, or the population in general, making it difficult to produce a medical protocol. Medically this is valid. However, that does not negate the efficacy of the therapy. It, instead points to the need for physicians of all types to focus on the patient and account for metabolic individuality when recommending treatment.

'It is better to know the person with the disease, than which disease the person has.' – Hippocrates

Even in ancient Greece, healers were recognizing the need to treat the individual as a whole rather than the disease as its own entity. It is time for physicians to get back to that practice and provide the healing that our patients are looking for.

Determining Food Allergies

Medical testing currently utilizes two methods of testing to determine food sensitivities, blood testing and a skin test called a Scratch Test, Skin Prick Test (SPT) or a puncture test. . I find the tests to be unreliable at best.

The blood test relies on markers in the blood to determine sensitivities. Since the blood is the very last to show pathology in the body, it serves as the final indication that there is a problem and not as an early indicator of malfunction. The blood will deplete other areas of the body to remain in balance so that we do not die. Because of this, the presence of dysfunction in the blood indicates end stage dysfunction which requires more work on the part of the body and the individual to correct.

The skin test is far less of an indicator. The potential allergens are injected into the epithelium of the skin and monitored for reaction. Metabolic reaction and epithelial reaction are not the same. The discovery that a substance irritates the substrates of the skin is not an accurate indicator of how the body will react when those substances are digested and brought into contact with the metabolic system.

In my office I use a method of testing developed by Dr. Donald Lapore called Muscle Response Testing (MRT), or Kinesiotesting. It relies on bio feedback from the body based on an energetic response to a substance.

Every living thing gives off energy and we all react to that energy. We can measure the energy with EEG's and

EKG's, we have even photographed it with Kirlian photography. Have you ever walked into a room and could feel when someone was in a bad mood? You are picking up on their energy. Ever stay in that room long enough that it puts you in a bad mood? That is your energy reacting to their energy. This is the basis of MRT.

Kinesiotesting is done by having the patient hold a vial of a substance up to the solar plexus while extending the other arm out to the side of the body. The tester then applies pressure to the extended arm with two fingers and tests for any change in resistance. A weakening of the ability to resist indicates a sensitivity to the substance in the vial. I measure on a scale of 1-5; 1 being no change in resistance and 5 being I can drop your arm with my pinky finger and no pressure. A baseline resistance is set at the beginning of the test to determine resistance ability and that individuals 1 setting. This test provides immediate and accurate bio feedback based on metabolic reaction since metabolism is primarily the production of and use of energy.

What Causes Food Allergies?

Nutritional Deficiency

Food allergies develop as a direct result of nutritional deficiency. Wheat in particular may be caused by a deficiency of EFA's, vitamin F, magnesium and the amino acid histidine.

Histidine is important in immune function as it is converted to histamine during an allergic reaction.

A fair amount of research has been done pointing to nutrient deficiency as the main cause of food allergies. As we saw earlier in Dr. Lapore's work, the deficiency of vitamins, minerals and amino acids contribute directly to the development of food allergies. However, other nutrient deficiencies may contribute to allergies. In *A Chemistry of Man*, Dr. Jensen states that "when oxygen is insufficient, digestion is poor and food is not assimilated properly; this encourages over eating because nourishment is needed."[7] Poor assimilation of foods leads to a lack of or imbalance in vitamins, minerals, and other nutrients. Dr. Lapore's findings support the link between nutrient imbalance and the development of food allergies, and so poor oxygen levels in the body may logically be linked to the development of food allergies. Dr. Ann Wigmore, discussed later in this book, stated that the deficiency of any one amino acid could result in the development of a food intolerance.

Immune Dysfunction

Immune dysfunction may be another cause; it may also be a by-product which contributes to further development of chronic disease. According to Naturalnews.com 'some food allergies cause body cells to swell (edema) leading to insulin resistance. Edema is a response to inflammation which contributes to a diabetic-type response in the body.'[8]

Immune response seems to be at the center of allergy manifestation in any patient. This is particularly true in the area of the brain responsible for immune function. Dr. Ballentine writes: "The hypothalamus is part of the 'circuit' that is active when one is anxious or upset. It is also the bridge to the pituitary gland which regulates the secretion of hormones." [9] Some of these hormones are important in the production and regulation of antibodies during immune response, as is the case during allergic reactions. Chronic allergic responses create ongoing inflammation and stimulating immune response. When the immune system is overly active, the body is constantly in defense mode. This state leaves little energy for repair. Without rest from defense, the organs may begin to malfunction as regular maintenance may be neglected by the body's repair mechanisms because nutrients and energy are tied up in the defense processes. The pancreas, for example, may shut down and cease to produce insulin, resulting in Type I diabetes. According to Naturalnews.com "Suspicion has fallen on diet as a trigger for Type I diabetes, which is usually diagnosed in childhood, following the surprise discovery that the condition is genetically similar to celiac disease, a gut disorder caused by intolerance to gluten, a protein found in wheat." [10]

Many persons battling chronic diseases have noted that during the holistic healing process, those foods which previously elicited and allergic response, ceased to be antagonistic to the body after a time. Anne Frahm stated that she was sensitive to tomatoes, but during her natural treatments to reverse her case of cancer, the sensitivity to tomatoes disappeared after some time of cleansing, detoxifying and nourishing her body with whole, live foods.[11] It is interesting to note that this phenomenon does to accompany allopathic treatments of chronic diseases, which is not surprising when one considers that allopathic medicine is very isolationist in its understanding of illness. The allopathic paradigm does not view the treatment of an illness as treatment of the entire person, but rather as the treatment of a specific organ or locus of the body without regard for the effects of the treatments upon the body as a whole. It focuses on symptom management rather than the elimination of the cause of the symptom(s).

By contrast, holistic medicine strives to focus directly on the return to health of the whole person with less regard for the disease. Support of the natural healing ability of the body is preferred over the treatment of defined disease. Vitamin and nutrition therapy is a prime example of this type of healing. The use of whole, raw, living foods to detoxify, cleanse and rejuvenate the body cannot isolate any one particular system with its effects. This is because the body is a complex, synergistic machine with all parts interdependently connected to maintaining vital processes as well as higher functions. It is also for this reason that it is unlikely that an individual would be lacking in only one nutrient, particularly with respect to the manifestation of food allergies.

Candida Albicans

It has been suggested that Candida Albicans may cause food sensitivities.[12] When this particular bacteria over runs the beneficial intestinal flora it can create perforations in the intestinal lining permitting the partially digested food to 'leak' from the gut into the blood stream, causing what has been diagnosed as leaky gut syndrome. These partially digest food particles have not been completely broken down into a form that is recognizable by the body. When they enter the blood stream, the body recognized the substance as 'foreign' and produces an immune response in the form of an allergy.

Devitalized Foods and GMO's

Another possibility is that the increased consumption of processed and refined foods which are stripped of nearly all usable nutrients in the refining process is creating severe nutrient deficiencies that are leading to food allergies.

Genetically modified organisms or GMO foods are also believed to be a possible cause of food allergies. The link between the rise of food allergies and the introduction of GMO foods into the general foods supply seem apparent when the facts are examined.

Beginning in 1994 a growing percentage of our food supply has come from products which have been genetically altered for one purpose or another. During that time the American population has experienced an increased occurrence of food allergies, irritable bowel syndrome and leaky gut syndrome.[13] According to interviewees in the documentary Genetic Roulette, changes in diet can correct food allergies.[14] One such person, Ashley Koff, RD, a registered dietitian claims that when she improves the quality of food for a patient by "prescribing" organic and non-GMO foods, the allergy symptoms go away and as the patient begins to heal, the allergen foods can again be consumed…"provided they are not GMO."[15]

The increased use of pesticides and herbicides in the production of our foods, by means of genetic modification to

30

produce plants that are resistant to herbicides and pesticides, is also suspected in the increased occurrence of food allergies. Increasing numbers of crops are produced with the aid of herbicides to control weeds and insecticides to manage crop damage from insects. Roundup is one such herbicide which is very prevalent in farming today. The main ingredient in this product is a chemical called glyphosate. Glyphosate manages weed production because it is a broad spectrum chelator.[16] Chelators chemically bond with micronutrients and make them biochemically unavailable to the organism during growth. These chemicals remain in the plant after harvest. When the plants are sprayed, the soil is saturated with the chemical along with the plant. As the plant takes up nutrients from the soil, it also absorbs more of the chemical herbicide and pesticide. This absorption from the soil increases the chemical concentration in the plant tissue. This cannot be removed by rinsing or washing the plant, it is then ingested when we consume the plant as food. Little direct evidence has been produced to directly the link this chemical to the manifestation of food allergies, but this theory appears to be a logical conclusion.

Associated Diseases

Many of the chronic diseases which have begun to occur with greater frequency over the past few decades are thought to be allergy based. As mentioned earlier, diabetes is possibly a result of unchecked food allergies. Chronic Fatigue, Colitis, Fibromyalgia, Adrenal Fatigue, IBS, Leaky Gut and migraine headaches are at the top of the list of disorders which may be caused, at least in part, by food intolerances or allergies.

Connection to Psychological Disorders.

There is another aspect of food allergy types that must be considered. While physical symptoms are typical of both food intolerances and anaphylactic allergies, the symptoms are not limited to epithelial or endothelial effects. Some symptoms may manifest in the mind. Cerebral allergies, which primarily affect the tissues of the brain, cause symptoms mirroring many psychological disorders. With the wide spread diagnosis of chronic disease and mental illness that we are witnessing today, we may find permanent relief from these maladies by simply identifying and correcting the underlying cause which is often based in food allergies.

Chapter 2

How Allergies Are Reversed

The reversal of food allergies, as with any chronic disease, is a three step process. In order to correct the allergies, we must first eliminate the cause of the allergies; toxicity and deficiency. Facilitating this healing requires us to boost the immune system, detoxify the body, and then repair damaged cells and regenerate dead cells.

Boosting the Immune System

Boosting or strengthening the immune system is a critical first step in reversing any disharmony or dis-ease in the body. This prepares the body for the work of flushing toxins out of the tissues and removing them from the body. Without a well-functioning immune system, the body can only eliminate toxins to the point at which toxicity can be removed from the body faster than the toxins are being introduced. When we reach that 'critical mass' point where the toxins are introduced faster than the body can eliminate them, this is the point at which the body can no longer adequately protect the body from those toxins. When we detox first, in the presence of chronic conditions, we do so with an impaired immune system. A weak or impaired immune system will give out during a detox. A fatigued immune system will not be able to protect the body from the onslaught of toxins and attackers that are pulled from the tissues during the detoxification process. As a result, we get 'knocked down' by the process and become ill. Beginning the reversal process by focusing on improving immune function, we are expanding the reach of the body to expel toxins.

How to Strengthen the Immune System

Boosting you immune system is a simple process. There are only five things needed to strengthen immune function.

Avoid foods and substances that are toxic or antagonistic to your body, eliminate sugary foods, caffeine products and allergen foods form the diet to allow your body to step out of defense mode, rest and give your immune cells to recharge.

Replace processed, packaged foods with whole, fresh, raw fruits and vegetables, whole grains, nuts, seeds and the like. Processed, packaged foods are any food which has gone through a manufacturing process that changes the lifespan or form of the food. If it has a nutritional label, it is a packaged food. Prior to being packaged, it had to be processed to give it an extended shelf-life – one that is longer than the food in its raw state. The processing cooks out enzymes and vital nutrients from the foods. In addition, preservatives and other chemical products are added to the food to enhance flavor and stabilize the product for its time in the plant, on the delivery truck, supermarket shelves and your pantry shelf prior to consumption. The process may also introduce synthetic replacement of the nutrients that were eliminated from the food during the manufacturing process. This applies to all packaged foods. A label that says 'No GMO' or 'Organic' on the package does not mean that it is more nutritious for you. It is still packaged and processed. It is also subject to the same FDA additive and preservative requirements as foods that do not have those labels.

Make sure that you are well hydrated. Your body needs water to regulate every system from higher brain function and memory function to digestion and waste elimination. Most Americans walk around dehydrated. To ensure that you are well hydrated, consume half of your body weight in ounces of water daily. In other words – take your current body weight, divide it in half. That is the number of ounces that you need to consume daily at a minimum to be adequately hydrated. Consume more if you are ill, active and during hot weather. There are only a few things that hydrate the body. Plain water is one. I recommend spring or artesian water because those types of waters have absorb nutrients via osmosis from the earth that they flow over or through. These waters are considered to be living waters because they contain natural forms of nutrients in a form that the body knows how to utilize. This type of water helps to balance minerals in the body as well as helping to maintain the proper level of alkalinity.

A Caution about Alkaline Waters

Avoid waters with gimmicks. Alkalized water is one of the popular examples of this. Alkalized water may initially alkalize an overly acidic body, but long term, it will result in a condition called alkalosis in which the body's pH is shifted too far to the alkaline side of the pH scale.

When the body is too alkaline, it can lead to confusion, dizziness, hand tremors, nausea, and vomiting, numbness or tingling in the face, hands and feet. It can also lead to prolonged muscle spasms. Extreme cases can lead to coma.

Another concern with this particular product is the method used to alkalize the water. Some manufacturers use sodium bicarbonate, commonly known as baking soda. Sodium bicarbonate destroys hemoglobin – the red protein in the blood responsible for transporting oxygen to the tissues.

Infused waters also hydrate the body. Infused waters are waters which have had raw fruits or vegetables slice up and soaked in the water without muddling or macerating the produce. Herbal teas are also considered infusions. These types of drinks give you a double health boost. Because the water is infused with the nutrients from the herbs or produce, we receive nutrition as well as hydration. Black teas , coffee, fizzy drinks, even sports drinks contain sugar, caffeine and other ingredients which chemically bond with the water molecule and cause the body to treat it as food. In addition, the sugar and other ingredients in those drinks trick our metabolism, leech water from the body and deplete us of vital nutrients.

Eat plenty of fruits and vegetables. I often advise my patients to put a rainbow of foods on their plate each meal. Start with a cup or more of dark green leafy vegetables, add in other vegetables in every color of the rainbow, and then round off the meal with a small portion of protein- 3-5 ounces is adequate. Creating your plate in this way ensures that you are getting all of the necessary nutrients at each meal because each color corresponds to a high amount of a certain nutrient. Yellow vegetables, for example, are high in magnesium and natural laxatives.

Finally, support your digestion by properly chewing your food and combining your foods correctly. In general, our society has established an 'eat on the go' policy that is counterproductive proper chewing and digestion in generals.

We should chew each bite until it is completely masticated and the consistency of tooth paste or creamy peanut butter. Chewing begins the digestive process by mixing in enzymes released into the saliva that start to break down the food before it leaves the mouth. Not chewing our food enough means that when the food reaches the stomach, it is not broken down far enough for the stomach to efficiently finish its portion of the digestive process and accounts, in part, for the development of that sluggish feeling that is referred to as food coma.

Improper combination of out foods is another factor in the development of the food coma feeling because the combination of some foods disrupts the digestive process and eliminates some important digestive tools. There are only four food combination rules. Following these rules will allow your digestion to function optimally, making the nutrients from your food fully available.

Rule #1. Consume fruits alone.

Fruits digest very quickly, taking approximately twenty minutes to make the trip through the entire digestive tract. Consuming fruits with slower digesting foods creates a traffic jam in the gut where the fruits continue to break down in the wrong area of the digestive system because they are stuck behind food that take longer to move through the digestive system. This can cause gassy, bloated feelings, belching and other such symptoms. It also creates the environment in the gut in which we reabsorb the toxic gases that are produced by the breakdown of the fruit that is not moving quickly enough through the gut. Wait 20 – 25 minutes after consuming fruits to eat another kind of food and at least 45 minutes after consuming all other types of food to eat fruits.

There are a few exceptions to this rule. Apples are one of the exception to this rule and may be combined with other foods. Dried fruits are another exception. Dried or dehydrated fruits lack the live enzymes of fresh fruits and therefore break down slower. My theory about why apples are an exception is that apples are actually a member of the herb family rather than a true fruit and the enzymes are active far longer than other fruits, making them digest slower.

Rule #2. Vegetables go with everything (except fruits).

Vegetables are the perfect companion for most other types of foods and provide the largest variety of nutrients. All vegetables contain carbohydrates, proteins and fats. Because of this, vegetables are most synergistic with other types of foods in providing us with vitamins as well as enzymes that are complementary in breaking down other foods.

Rule #3. DO NOT combine proteins and starches.

This rule is often one of the hardest for Americans to follow because this is what the typical American meal looks like: a meat, a starch and maybe a small portion of colorful vegetables. Protein foods include any animal product – meat, fish, dairy and eggs- as well as beans, lentils and other legumes. Starch foods are going to be your white foods – white potatoes, grains, breads, pastas, rice, etc.

When we consume a protein, our body produces an enzyme that breaks them down. When we consume a starch, our body produces another enzyme that breaks down those foods. When we consume proteins and starches together, both enzymes are released at the same time and they neutralize each other. Under these circumstances, no amount of chewing will break down those foods to the point they should be digested for the stomach to receive them and finish the digestive process because the tools needed to facilitate early digestion in the mouth are absent. This action can result in the heavy, sluggish feeling that many get after eating and is, in part, the reason most of us feel as though we need a nap after eating our Thanksgiving meal.

If you consume a protein, have it with a vegetable. If you eat a starch, have it with a vegetable. Wait at least 45 minutes after consuming a protein to eat a starch and vice versa.

Rule #4. DO NOT drink with your meals.
Drinking with our meals dilutes the gastric juices, weakening them. These weaker stomach acids do not break down our foods as efficiently as the full strength ones. Consuming up to two ounces of <u>any type</u> of liquid is acceptable, any more than that will disrupt your digestive process. Optimally, stop consuming liquids 30 minutes prior eating and wait 30 minutes after finishing your food to drink anything.

In addition to producing lethargy and other gastric symptoms, improper food combination also results in excessive consumption of energy and makes that energy unavailable to the rest of the body for functions such as cleansing, repair and regeneration.

Applying these five simple rules for 3-4 weeks prior to detoxing will allow your immune system to rest and recharge.

1. Avoid metabolic antagonists
2. Replace packaged processed foods with whole foods
3. Stay hydrated
4. Eat the rainbow in vegetables
5. Support your digestion

Detoxification

Detoxification is a necessary step in reversing any disease. The body must be free of toxins that produce an immune response in order to permit the body to concentrate its energy on repair rather than defense. No healing can be affected by any substance which affects the body in such a way that it must expend more energy on defense than on repair. The constant introduction of toxic substances from inorganic food preservatives or growth chemicals as well as lifestyle contaminates such as tobacco, alcohol and drugs including prescription and over the counter drugs, chemical household products and allergen producing foods create an ongoing state of defensive action by the body.

A well designed, implemented and managed detoxification program allows the body to 'hit the reset button' and when followed up with proper dietary and lifestyle changes, produces rapid, sustainable healing. It is for this reason that we implement a detoxification program in the reversal of any food allergy, as with any state of dis-ease. The details of the detoxification plan vary slightly from individual to individual.

This variance is to account for the biochemical differences inherent in the individual.

The premise, objective and structure of the detoxification program remain the same, only the food choices change, based on individual constitution and need. The length of detoxification required also varies based on individual need. Duration of detoxification ranges from two to thirty days with an average duration of seven days.

The detoxification program in my clinical study consisted of a strict regimen of a live juice fast for no less than two days and not more than seven days and reasonable elimination of lifestyle and environmental toxins as well as the use of herbal teas and enemas, where appropriate. The details of a generic detoxifying regimen are available in Appendix A. Each participant also completed a food journal for the duration of the study.

Following the detoxification each participant consumed a diet of whole, live, mostly raw fruits and vegetables consumed at regular intervals throughout the day to ensure that blood glucose levels remain steady and in participants avoid creating an internal environment which recreates inflammation due to spikes and drops in blood sugar. Live juices continued to be consumed to supplement meals as maintenance for a period of no less than 30 days and continuing through the duration of the study in cases of severe malnutrition.

As was deemed appropriate based on MRT responses in to all allergen groups with a score of 1 consistently for two weeks, the allergy producing foods were reintroduced and reactions recorded. Each allergy producing food was reintroduced first in its organic, non-GMO form and then in the GMO form in order to determine the role of GMO foods in producing food allergies and intolerances.

Repair and Regeneration

As discussed previously, all chronic degenerative diseases, including food allergies, are caused by two things – toxicity and deficiency. When the body is too toxic to absorb nutrients, it becomes deficient. This deficiency makes the body unable to keep up with the demand to rid the body of toxins. This begins a cycle of toxins overrunning the body, depleting the body further of nutrients which perpetually repeats until the cycle is actively stopped.

Once the body has been detoxified, the process of repairing the body begins almost simultaneously. The removal of toxins from the body frees up energy that was previously spent on defense to be redirected into repair of damaged cells and regeneration of necrotic ones. This process does not happen overnight, but is does happen faster than you think. It talks about three months for a cell to regenerate. The only need for regeneration to occur, is that all of the necessary building blocks be present in appropriate quantities and that the required construction team be available to the body.

The building blocks of the body are nutrients; vitamins, minerals, amino acids, oxygen and water. The construction team is comprised of various enzymes which 'demo' old, damaged and necrotic cells, and then use the nutrients to rebuild replacement cells or repair the damaged ones.

Earlier we discussed the food combination rules. Repair relies on adhering to those rules. We must consume foods that are rich in all of those nutrients in order to heal and remain well. Proper food combinations and proportions are essential for healing because consuming food types disproportionately to what is optimal for your body requires the body to work harder to break down and utilize the foods and limit the variety of nutrients that you have access to metabolically. Improper food combination disrupts the digestion process and employs additional energy to breakdown and assimilate the usable nutrients in those foods.

Eliminating Animal Products

With most patients, animal products are eliminate from the diet for a time. The elimination of meats, dairy, eggs and fish from the individual's diet allows the digestion to expend less energy.

Animal products are a source of protein because they are flesh. All flesh is comprised of a chain of amino acids. Human, chicken, beef, fish or other animal flesh are all made of proteins. Each protein has a specific configuration of amino acids chemically bonded to create that protein. These protein chains are not the same across species lines, a fish protein, for example, is not the same configuration of amino acids as a beef protein or chicken protein. No animal protein has the same chemical configuration as a human protein molecule. In order for our body to utilize the protein from animal flesh, we must break the chemical bond of the protein molecule to free the individual amino acids. We must then extract the amino acids that we need, then combine them with the amino acids that our body produces in order to

44

create a human protein. Since breaking a chemical bond requires more energy than that required to create a bond, eliminating animal products from the diet allows the body to use less energy for digestion and redirect the energy that would have been used to break down the animal protein into healing.

Acidic Ash

Some foods create an acidic ash inside the body when burned off in the metabolic process. This ash shifts the internal pH of the body to the acidic side of the scale. Becoming too acidic will kill us. When our body's pH becomes acidic, an immune response is initiated to protect the body from the danger. Sugary, starchy, and animal based foods produce the highest amounts of this kind of metabolic ash.

To avoid creating an internal environment that is overly acidic, these types of foods should be consumed rarely.

The Benefits of Raw Food

Living foods are the basis of vitamin and nutrition therapy. With this type of treatment, the body is receiving all of the nutrients required to maintain, detoxify and repair the body. A living food is any food that still contains the active enzymes and other nutrients in their natural state. These quickly disintegrate as the food finishes its life process and begins to die. The fruit or vegetable begins to die as soon as it is harvested from the plant. Fresh, whole fruits and vegetables, raw nuts, seeds, legumes and whole grains in their natural state are classified as living foods. These foods are still vital and contain all of the nutrients needed for a healthy body. We are vital, living beings. The chronic consumption of dead, devitalized, nutrient void foods leads us to become nutrient deficient, devitalized beings, a state which, when left uncorrected, leads to disease and, eventually, death.

In my clinic, I am constantly recommending that patients consume fruits and vegetables as close to 'off the plant' as possible to ensure that they are consuming the most vital living foods. These foods are full of all of the necessary building blocks, especially the living enzymes. Living foods ideally make up 80% or more of a vitalizing diet, grains make up an additional 10%, with animal products making up 10% or less of the diet. Sugary, refined, and processed foods should be consumed rarely.

Why this works

This type of therapy works because it not only addresses the underlying cause of the allergies, but is also honors the basic natural healing principals. Those principals recognize that the body knows how to be well, it is designed to be in a state of balance called homeostasis. The body will go to extreme measures to maintain this homeostasis and all of the mechanisms are already in place to bring the body back into balance when necessary so long as we provide the body with the right fuel and building blocks and then get out of our own way.

Consider what happens when we get a cut on our arm. What do you really need to do in order to ensure that your injury heals? All that is necessary is that we keep the wound clean and leave it alone, the body does the rest. The same is true of every part of the body.

The ability of the body to heal does not rely on products or innovative medical procedures or pharmaceuticals. It relies on something far more sophisticated, a mechanism that was designed to rebalance itself and re-harmonize its internal workings- the human body.

Maintenance

Maintaining a healthy body is equally as simple as rebuilding the damaged body. Adhering to the 80/20 rule and performing periodic maintenance detoxification are all that are required to avoid the recurrence of disease.

The 80/20 rule states that if we are providing our bodies with the appropriate nutrients in the right proportion and the right combinations 80% of the time, then the body can handle the 20% of the junk that we throw at it. Implementing this rule means that you can enjoy social events with family and friends without feeling guilty about indulging in foods that are less than optimal or even useless in nourishing the body.

Maintenance detoxing need not be an elaborate ordeal. Simply taking a couple of days, several times a year to consume nothing but live, whole fresh fruits and vegetables provides the body the opportunity and tools to 'reset'. If you are adhering to the 80/20 rule, the body will not be overly toxic and the detoxification process will on strain the immune system. This means that the work that must be done at the beginning of a healing process does not need to be repeated during maintenance because you are consistently providing the body with all that is needed to keep the immune system strong.

The work that I am doing at my clinic with food allergies and other chronic degenerative diseases is not new, many others have done this same work successfully. In the next chapter, I will discuss some of the forerunners in vitamin and nutrition therapy.

Chapter 4

Building on Previous Studies and Successes

Throughout the last century the study of food allergies along with many other chronic degenerative diseases has resulted in very important discoveries which are especially important to holistic healers. Dr. Max Gerson, Dr. Ann Wigmore, Dr. Donald Lapore, and most recently Dr. Michael Savage have contributed to the findings on this subject. While much of these doctors' works overlap, there are some significant methods and discoveries which are unique to each of them. It is upon an eclectic approach based on the significant work of each of these pioneers that I have based my own research.

Dr. Gerson's work

Dr. Max Gerson worked extensively with chronic degenerative diseases. His methods are primarily based on vitamin and nutrition therapies. During his time he successfully cured migraines, diabetes, rare skin diseases and, most reputably, cancers of all kinds. He was his own first patient, curing himself of migraines as a young physician. His self-treatment began by ingesting copious amounts of freshly prepared apple juice and other apple preparations, which he termed 'the apple diet'. He later slowly added other foods, one food at a time. During this process he noticed that when a particular food did not agree with him, he would develop a migraine headache in as few as twenty minutes.[17] This may have been one of the first correlations drawn between migraine headaches and food allergy.

Further on in his career he cured Dr. Albert Schweitzer of diabetes, Mrs. Schweitzer of skin tuberculosis- a form of lupus, and Dr. Schweitzer's daughter of a rare, unnamed skin disease. Again he accomplished this by first administering freshly prepared fruit and vegetable juice along with a vegetarian diet of both raw and cooked foods.

The Gerson Therapy has successfully treated a wide range of health problems. In addition to the conditions listed above, addictions, epilepsy, macular degeneration and liver cirrhosis have been successfully corrected on the therapy. Allergies were successfully reversed along with chronic fatigue syndrome, Chrohn's disease, and colitis, all of which are believed to be allergy based.[18]

He believed that there was a link between the foods that we consume and the health of our bodies. While, today, this is not necessarily profound, it was, at the time, paramount to the revolution of nutritional healing. His approach was based on the paradigm that the body is capable of healing itself provided the correct building blocks are available to the body. These building blocks are the necessary nutrients provided in the correct balance to nourish the body and reverse the disease process. This therapy consists of the use of 'liberal amounts of high-quality nutrition... improving one's depressed immune system.'[19] This was accomplished with the use of fresh vegetable and fruit juices, whole raw and cooked vegetarian diet and the addition of specific vitamin supplements.

Dr. Gerson placed a specific emphasis on hyper-nutrating because deficiency in the body contributes to degenerative disease development.[20] He particularly believed that the lack of oxygen prohibits the body from eliminating toxins, eventually leading to the development of many diseases. The process of introducing large quantities of necessary nutrients to the patient increased the oxygen available for use within the metabolic processes of the body thus strengthening immune defenses.

The use of live or freshly prepared fruit and vegetable juices remains paramount to The Gerson Therapy. In order to introduce into the body sufficient quantities of nutrients to facilitate and expedite healing, one would need to consume in excess of 17 pounds of whole food daily. This feat would be difficult for even the most veracious appetite. To ensure that each patient could accommodate such large quantities of nutrients from food sources, Dr. Gerson utilized freshly juiced fruits and vegetables consumed by the patient before the juice began to breakdown and loose enzymes and other nutrients (usually within two hours of juicing) vital to the recovery of the patient. By removing the indigestible fiber from the fruits and vegetables and consuming the remaining juice, the patient is able to consume far more nutrients than could reasonably be consumed and processed in a single day from whole foods alone. In addition, the removal of the pulp allows faster bioavailability of the nutrients and easier absorption in the small intestines. This process also frees up energy that would have been used in the digestive process and allows it to be redirected to repair and regeneration of cells. Patients on Dr. Gerson's therapy protocol often consumed 8 oz. of fresh juice each waking hour in addition to the prescribed whole vegetarian foods.

Whole, fresh vegetarian foods are included as part of the protocol in order to maintain proper digestive flora and provide the necessary ingredients to ensure that eliminative processes are not disrupted. The patient is fed three nutritious meals per day of mostly raw whole vegetarian foods along with 8 ounces of fresh juice every hour beginning at 8 am until 7pm. [21]

Finally, very specific vitamin supplements were added to The Gerson Therapy. These supplements consisted of potassium salts, thyroid, Lugol's iodine solution, pancreatic enzymes, and niacin as well as medical injections with vitamin B12.[22] All of these protocols were used to accomplish three things for the patient:[23]

- Harmonize the person's biochemistry
- Elevate the workings of a suppressed immune system
- Correct the malfunctioning of essential organs

Dr. Gerson stated that "all chronic degenerative diseases respond positively to vitamin and nutrition therapy because invariably they are caused by two things; toxicity and deficiency."[24] When the body becomes toxic and unable to rid itself of the build up quickly enough to keep up with the demand placed on it by the introduction of toxins, the body becomes saturated and clogged. It then has difficulty properly processing and assimilating nutrients in the foods consumed, becoming deficient. This creates a vicious cycle of chronic toxicity and ongoing nutrient deficiency. This is especially true in instances where the diet is deficient in the required nutrients from the beginning, as with the Standard American

Diet. When we eliminate the toxicity, we produce an environment in which the body is more easily able to procure and utilize the nutrients from foods. The introduction then of whole, fresh foods to the body promotes both the detoxification of the body as well as supplying the necessary nutrients to correct deficiency and reverse the disease process. The application of this particular principle is helpful in correcting food allergies.

Dr. Wigmore's work

Dr. Ann Wigmore's work has been of less influence than other forerunners in the area of reversing food allergies, but the theories and practices in her work still merit a review. While her focus was primarily on the cure of cancer, she also found distinct correlations between toxicity in the body and the development of food allergies. Her therapy, which centers on detoxification of the body and the use of wheatgrass juice to reintroduce nutrients to the body, has been effective in facilitating the healing process for many chronic degenerative diseases. Dr. Wigmore noted that the deficiency of just one amino acid could result in an allergy. [25] This is confirmed by Dr. Lapore, who identified deficiency of specific amino acids contributing to allergic reactions to specific groups foods.

Wheatgrass is described as a complete food because of its chlorophyll content. Chlorophyll contains a very balanced ratio of all of the necessary organic mineral salts, vitamins and all eight essential amino acids. For this reason, wheatgrass is viewed by Dr. Wigmore and her contemporaries as a super food. As such the juice of this plant was the primary source of nutrition and detoxification in Dr. Wigmore's therapy.

Through her experiences, both clinical and personal, she came to believe that wheatgrass juice helped the body to rid itself of waste products and toxins which had accumulated in tissues and cells of the body. She also believed that years of choosing foods which lacked proper nutritional balance and where loaded with chemical preservatives eventually this would cause the filtration system in the body to reach a "critical mass" point at which it begins to break down and manifest disease. This 'breaking point' makes cleansing necessary in order for the body to begin healing. The following excerpt sums up Dr. Wigmore's approach to healing.

> Ann Wigmore believed cell toxemia, from nutritional deficiency and stresses, is the only disease in western man. Toxemia is a word used to explain poisons that are stored in the body. Over toxicity is created by eating processed, unnatural, and chemical laden foods and having a body that is not optimally flushing out these toxins.

> Ann Wigmore taught that the body can help to *release* these stored poisons by feeding it living foods, with plenty of enzymes that are easy to digest.

> Once the body eliminates stored toxins and poisons that have accumulated in the blood stream and colon, the cells are able to receive nourishment, thus enabling the immune system to strengthen and rebuild.

Poor health is a manifestation from the body losing its ability to digest foods and absorb nutrients. Deficiency disorders are thus created, including allergies which are so prevalent today.[26]

The method utilized to correct food allergies was essentially the same as the methods she used for the correction of any other disease.

'She found consuming wheatgrass juice, raw

foods and sprouts, performing exercise, having

peace of mind and a positive emotional state to

be what would bring one closest to finding the

"fountain of youth." [27]

In her book, _Naturama Living Textbook_, Dr. Wigmore states "Every incurable health problem… should be handled in the same manner: by cleansing the blood stream and taking care of deficiencies, the body will be able to heal the problem. Every person can help themselves and frankly, it is only through their own efforts, through the efforts their bodies make, that healing takes place and health and youth return."[28]

In the late 1950's and early 1960's Dr. Wigmore, together with Viktoras Kluvinskas, began The Hippocrates Institute where she put into practice the healing methods which she used herself to regain health. The main stay of this therapy was the use of living foods and fresh wheatgrass juice. A diet exclusively of freshly juiced wheatgrass, as well as fruits and vegetables, sprouts, seeds and nuts in their raw form was used by Dr. Wigmore and her colleagues to successfully heal patients.

Dr. Wigmore was one of the earliest proponents of the raw or living food diet in which a person consumes only those foods which are still alive (containing active enzymes) when consumed. Such foods as fresh, whole fruits and vegetables consumed as close to 'fresh off the plant' as possible, raw nuts and seeds, legumes and sprouts from vegetables, beans and seeds would be included on this diet. This particular approach to food, as it applies to healing, has proven to be very effective.

Even though her work heavily incorporated diet, she is best known as the pioneer of wheat grass juicing. Her method of extraction the live juice from the freshly harvested blades of wheat grass is still considered the most optimal method. Fresh clippings of the grass are cut from a personal crop of the plant (which may be grown indoor and cultivated year round as well as hydroponically). The juice is then extracted from the clippings by inserting the entire bunch into a masticating juice extractor which 'chews' the clippings and squeezes out the juice, simultaneously separating the pulp. It is recommended that the juice be combined with other fresh fruit and vegetable juices and consumed with in a few hours of preparation. Daily consumption is also recommended for maximum benefit.

Evidence certainly exists as to the efficacy of the therapeutic use of wheat grass juice. While most such evidence is considered anecdotal, the persons whom have benefited from the application of this therapy probably do not feel that the results are unproven. Administering just 100mL per day to patients with acute, active ulcerative colitis in a double blind study produced noted improvement in those receiving the wheat grass juice. Symptoms worsened in those patients receiving the placebo.[29]

It is believed to be the enzymes and chlorophyll content in wheat grass which provide the necessary nutrients to facilitate healing in the body; the plant contains nearly 70% chlorophyll by most accounts. Wheat grass juice has been used in the successful treatment diabetes, colitis, burns, skin ulcers, arthritis, and arteriosclerosis as well as cases of eczema and nasal congestion.[30] The nutrients in chlorophyll are not exclusive to wheat grass. These nutrients are abundant in all dark green leafy vegetables. Foods like kale, chard, spinach and all other types of greens contain high quantities of chlorophyll and essential amino acids.

Dr. Savage's work

Dr. Michael Savage is most well known as a political talk show host and author of politically oriented books, but he has also authored at least 15 books on nutrition and natural healing. In his writing, he speaks very frankly about the disease trap that we can fall into when we disregard the laws of nature and the natural function of the body. In _Healing Children Naturally_, Dr. Savage discusses ways in which doctors may identify food allergies including the _empirical diet_.

An interesting point that he made in this book was regarding food preferences in young children. He suggests that a child's dislike of specific foods may be an instinctual mechanism by which the child avoids foods that produce allergic responses in his or her body. [31]

Accidental introduction of allergen foods into the body is common place in the typical American diet since it is primarily made up of processed and refined foods which may contain offending foods as fillers or list them under more scientific names which are misleading to the average consumer. Wheat, eggs, milk and soy are the most difficult to avoid as some derivative of these foods is present in nearly all processed and packaged foods. Because it is so difficult to avoid allergens when consuming processed foods, Dr. Savage advocates a diet of whole fresh fruits and vegetables as well as meats and dairy when those foods do not create allergic reactions in the individual. Elimination & desensitization diets as well as herbal preparations of passion flower are recommended by Dr. Savage for the treatment of food sensitivities.[32]

Migraines are another condition which is believed to be brought on by food allergies in some cases. The unexpected onset of migraines, especially in children, may be caused by food allergies. Among the common offenders here are dairy, chocolate, nuts, wheat, meats, and chemical additives, especially color additives.[33]

Many individuals with anaphylactic reactions to foods indicate that migraines are among the symptoms experienced just before or after an attack. In my personal experience, the use of epinephrine to counter an anaphylactic reaction to nuts alleviated airway constriction, but intensified migraine headaches and the accompanying nausea. In contrast, the use of an herbal tincture preparation of Osha Root eliminated all symptoms of anaphylaxis with no development of migraine or related symptoms.

Dr. Savage recommends withholding all foods at first, with the exception of fruit juices and herbal teas from non-allergenic sources. Follow this with an elimination diet to identify the allergy. Headaches may be treated with herbal teas of balm, lavender, or guto kola.

Ulcerative Colitis is a relatively recent addition to the many diagnoses of intestinal disorders. It may have its origins in food intolerances as well. The immune response to the antagonistic food takes place during the digestive process where extra mucus is secreted to protect the tissues from harm by the 'invader'. This mucus is then passed from the body through the colon with or without stool. Usually the mucus is accompanied by blood which may be caused by the introduction of foods into the small intestines that have not been properly alkalized after leaving the stomach. This exposes the small intestines to very acidic materials, possibly eroding the intestinal lining and creating bleeding ulcers along the intestinal tract. This condition can be progressive and depletes the body of vast amounts of nutrients, leading to nutritional deficiency as well as severe dehydration.

Dr. Savage's approach to healing this condition is less focused on reversing the food allergies which may initially cause it and more is directly focused on ensuring that the body receives appropriate nutrients. Since the condition "tends to resolve itself spontaneously"[34], Dr. Savage recommends a high calorie diet with large amounts of protein and high vitamin & mineral content, but with few starchy carbohydrates. The diet should consist of mainly foods which produce low residue such as cooked-pureed fruits and vegetables, fruit and vegetable juices, cottage cheese, bouillon and broths. [35] Red raspberry or Spanish chestnut herbal preparations may be used to control the diarrhea.

In my practice, identifying the presence of allergies or intolerances is one of the many test performed during the patients first visit to determine the underlying cause of any symptom. Using Kinesiotesting, I am able to immediately determine if a food or group of foods is antagonistic. Those foods can then be immediately eliminate from the diet with the confidence that those foods are the culprit. This allows us to speed the healing process along.

Dr. Lapore's Work

Dr. Donald Lapore's work has been most influential with regard to non-invasive diagnostic methods to determine which allergies are present in a patient as well as the correlation between nutritional imbalances and the development of those allergies. It is for this reason that the author is including more detailed information regarding Dr. Lapore's work.

Dr. Lapore determined that food intolerances or *metabolic antagonists*, as he called them, were a result of a nutritional imbalance. A deficiency of specific vitamins, minerals or amino acids would create a response from the body to certain foods which manifests the symptoms consistent with those of allergies.[36] This opinion was not held by only him.

According to Dr. Jensen, a deficiency of pantothenic acid causes incomplete or defective digestion which can produce food allergies ranging from mild intolerances to violent reactions.[37] Many of the allergies identified by Dr. Lapore reference one or more B vitamin deficiency as a contributing factor. He found that certain foods could be grouped together into categories of allergens and tested for these groups accordingly. These groups are depicted in Table 1-1.

He also recognized that some food allergies where common in individuals who also suffered from environmental allergies leading him to the discovery that nutritional deficiencies also effected the development of allergies other than those to food. Patients testing positive for wheat allergies often suffered from hay fever, animal dander allergies, and other chemical or environmental sensitivities.

Dr. Lapore devised a method of testing a person for such intolerances using Applied Kinesiology or Muscle Response Testing (MRT also called Kinesiotesting) and began helping patients eliminate their food intolerances using nutritional supplements and dietary changes. His testing method determined deficiencies in specific vitamins and minerals. This testing accomplishes three things; it identifies the allergy, measures the needed nutritional remedy or *nutritional antidote* necessary to reverse the allergy and measures needed support nutrients. These support nutrients act as catalysts for the nutritional antidote and aid in its absorption.[38] A nutritional antidote may be a vitamin, mineral, amino acid, herb or homeopathic remedy.[39]

To test a person using Dr. Lapore's MRT method, one should stand facing the patient. Once this is done, have the patient hold their non-dominant arm out to the side and press down on the outstretched arm using only two fingers placed approximately ½ inch above the wrist. Do this first with no activation of acupoints and with the patient holding nothing. This initial 'test' sets a baseline for the patient's ability to resist and allows the patient to feel how much pressure will be applied. At this point active testing may begin. Do this by place one vial of an allergen substance in the patient's dominant hand and have the patient hold the substance to the solar plexus (the area of the abdomen just above the navel where the lower ribs make an inverted 'v') and press down on the non-dominant arm again using only two fingers. Repeat this process for each allergen that you wish to test. Nutrients are tested similarly. Rather than having the patient hold the nutrient, acupoints are pressed by the patient while pressure is applied to measure resistance. * I use a scale of 1-5 to rate the changes in resistance. 1 being no change in resistance and five being – I can drop your arm with my pinky finger and no pressure. Typically at the 4-5 range we begin to see the development of severe allergic reaction and other chronic diseases.

Determining the necessary dose of any nutrient is accomplished by first testing for the deficiency as described above. Next place capsules of the nutrient in the patients hand as with allergies and testing, then adding additional amounts of the nutrient to the patient's hand until the resistance in the patient's arm does not vary from the base line when it is pressed. It is important to inform the patient

---

* MRT may be used to determine weakness in specific organs as well. This is useful in pinpointing which organs may require additional support in all forms of healing.

to keep the tongue away from the roof of the mouth during all testing because the tongue touching the roof of the mouth disrupts the bioelectric signal to acupoints and will render the test inaccurate. [40]

Once allergens have been identified and the proper dose of antidote is established, the healing process is quite simple. The patient is instructed to take the necessary antidote(s) while avoiding the antagonists for four days, returning on the fifth day for retesting and adjustment to antidotes if necessary. This process of testing, antidote(s), and retesting continues until the patient tests negative for the allergen(s).[41]

In my practice, I do not use supplements. Instead, the patient is given a regimen of whole foods and proper hydration in order to prepare the immune system for the detoxification process. I also instruct the patient to eliminate all allergen foods from his or her diet until the body has become rebalanced.

This particular practice is used because I am never exclusively working to reverse food intolerances. It is very rare to see someone in my office who only exhibits food allergy symptoms. It is nearly always necessary to work diligently work to reverse the cause of all disease: toxicity and nutritional deficiency.

Chapter 5

A Summary of a Clinical Study of Food Intolerance Responses to Whole Food and Vitamin/Mineral Therapy.

Parameters of the study

A 90 day clinical study of the effectiveness of reversing food allergies and intolerances with vitamin and nutrition therapy was conducted with volunteers. The goal was to provide conclusive evidence as to the link between nutritional and environmental agents in causing food allergies and intolerances as well as the viability in reversing the allergies through the use of vitamin and natural nutrition therapy. Reintroduction of allergen foods into the diet of the participant with lessened or absences of reaction were the indicators of success. Using Dr. Lapore's MRT, each participant was tested for food allergies as well as vitamin and mineral deficiencies upon beginning the study. Results were recorded on a scale of 1 to 5; 1 indicating no change in resistance from the baseline, and 5 indicating that there was no ability to resist pressure when applied. This scale was used in all MRT testing throughout out the study for continuity. Based on the results of these tests a customized diet and supplement plan was designed for each participant. This plan was adjusted weekly after retesting to ensure that nutrients were not inadvertently swung to the opposite spectrum creating additional imbalance. Weekly retesting marked the progress of each participant and was used as a gage for determining when to reintroduce allergen foods. The use of Dr. Lapore's MRT method was the primary diagnostic method used in determining nutritional needs; however, his use of isolate supplements was not implemented in this study. The approach to correcting the nutritional imbalances was a combination of whole-raw- live foods, live juices and herbal supplements as required by each participant. Herbs, primarily in the form of teas were implemented as part of the early morning routine for most participants.

Each participant was required to strictly follow a diet and supplement regimen designed specifically for his/her unique bio chemistry and allergy needs. Restrictions to diet and lifestyle habits varied from participant to participant and included smoking cessation, abstention from alcohol, abstention from illicit or recreational drugs and alterations to prescription medication as approved by attending physicians

Failure to adhere strictly to the program requirements disqualified participants from further participation as deviation from the program adds additional factors into the study and had the potential to skew the data.

This study was a continuation of the work already established by Doctors Gerson, Cousin, Lapore, Wigmore and Savage. These pioneers have been reversing minor allergies for decades with the use of food and vitamins. Our study took, for the first time, a close look at the efficacy of these same therapies for the complete reversal of minor allergies as well as anaphylactic producing allergies.

Methods Used to Determine Metabolic Support Requirements during Treatment

Thorough examination of each participant was conducted upon commencement of the study. Blood type[42] as well as metabolic type was used to determine optimal nutritional components for each participant.† Blood type is important in selecting those foods which will be most beneficial to revitalizing the individual's health. However, there are other factors in biochemical make up which must be considered. Since a person's genetic blood type may be a dominant gene with a recessive component, determining metabolic type allows the physician to identify recessive components of the genetic makeup which may be dominating the metabolic process. It is especially important to determine metabolic type for 'A' blood types and 'AB' blood types, because both have multiple blood type genes as factors.

An 'A' blood type individual, like everyone else, receives one blood type gene from one parent and another blood type gene from the other parent. A true 'A' blood type receives an A blood type gene from each parent, however, this rarely happens. Most often the individual receives an 'A' gene from one parent and an 'O' gene from the other. This genetic combination results in an 'Ao' genotype where, when tested, the antibodies for 'A' are present, but the 'O' blood type gene, which is recessive, dominates the metabolic process. There is no direct test to determine this genetic type without testing the individual's parents. However, we can determine

---

† Metabolic type testing is the work of Isabella de la Rosa; however the correlation between blood types and metabolic types with regard to metabolic dominance is the authors own work based on observations and work both personal and clinical.

if these factors exist by testing the individual for his or her metabolic type.

'A' blood types do very well on vegan diets. An 'A' Blood type person can survive much longer in a meat deprived environment (and often will thrive) than can an 'O' blood type which metabolically requires some animal product. When 'A' blood types eat animal products, feelings of lethargy ensue as well as those of sluggishness and mental fogginess. This is an indication that the food consumed is very difficult for his or her body to process and assimilate, requiring more energy to be drawn by the digestive system. This energy is pulled from high body functions to accommodate the additional requirements of the digestive system. This, however, does not always occur in 'A' blood types. When an 'A' blood type tests as a Protein metabolic type, it is an almost definite indicator that the individual is in fact an 'Ao' type and that the recessive 'O' gene is dominating the individual's metabolic processes.

This is true with 'AB' blood types as well. Since 'A' and 'B' genes are equally dominant, a person receiving one 'A' gene and one 'B' gene will test as an 'AB' blood type. In order to determine which gene is dominating metabolic processes, it is helpful to determine the metabolic type of the individual. As stated previously, 'A' blood types do very well on vegan diet and 'O' blood types require animal products, but, 'B' blood types is middle of the road doing very well on diets which are primarily plant based and those which include animal products.

Like blood type, there are a limited number of metabolic types which a person may be classified. Carb types require far less protein in the diet than the other metabolic types and often do well on diets completely devoid of animal products. Protein types as the name implies, require larger portions of protein to thrive and often require some animal product. Mixed types are a mix of the Carb and Protein type requirements and most often require an equal ratio of carbohydrates and proteins. Mixed metabolic types are very well adapted to process protein from both plant and animal sources. Because metabolic type does is not linked to a specific gene, it is much simpler to determine based on personal preferences and the responses of one's body to food choices. A simple 25 question test was used to determine each participant's metabolic type.

The methods used to determine nutrient deficiency allow us to identify these weaknesses before any deficiencies can be detected via lab work in the blood. This is because the blood is the last of the internal systems to manifest pathology.

Iris analysis or iridology, a diagnostic method is used to determine at which stage manifested inflammation is, and, on subsequent visits, the degree of healing taking place. Iridology is also based on the same principal as reflexology in that areas of the eye 'reflect' the condition of other parts of the body.

Sample Size

The initial sample group consisted of 21 participants suffering from food intolerances/allergies. Most participants were aware of the specific foods which produced allergic reaction prior to coming on to the study, however, each tested positive for multiple food allergies. None of the participants were aware of all of the food allergies for which he or she tested positive. Those with anaphylactic allergies also tested positive for multiple food intolerances. Participants were separated into two groups.

Group I consisted of 18 individuals with food intolerances presenting no life threatening symptoms of diverse ethnic and socioeconomic backgrounds, both male and female with ages ranging from 22 to 45. Some of the participants also presented with other complicating factors including; Type II diabetes, glaucoma, high blood pressure, high cholesterol, depression, reproductive system complications, sleep apnea, hypothyroidism, cholectomy, IBS and fallacemia.

Group II included 3 individuals with food intolerances which produced life threatening symptoms of diverse ethnic and socioeconomic backgrounds. All of the members of this group were female between the ages of 35 and 45. Other complicating factors for members of this group included Type II diabetes, pre-diabetes, reproductive system complications, sleep apnea, hypothyroidism, and cholectomy. All of the members of this group also presented low immune function.

Method
Over the course of this study, each participant was given a weekly meal plan which included recipes and specific instructions for food preparation and interval of food consumption.
All junk foods, processed and refined foods were a strictly eliminated. Participants were instructed to consume only organic, fresh fruits and vegetables, nuts, seeds, legumes and whole grains in which the natural enzymes of the plants were still active at the time of consumption and whole foods with minimal cooking. *Nutritional isolates* where not used in this

study as the purpose of this study was to prove the efficacy of reversing food allergies with living, whole foods and vitamins.

Live juices were important sources of necessary nutrients for the participants and were used in lieu of isolate supplements, where necessary. The live juices provided not only nutrients in larger quantities than could be consumed with the whole foods alone, but also the active enzymes of those foods which are not available in nutritional isolates.

Reintroduction of allergen foods was administered two fold, first with non-GMO foods and then again with commercial foods.

Results from the clinical study

Final sample size and demographics

Only five of the original participants completed the entire 12 weeks (90 days) of the study. Nine did not return after week 1, four exited after week 2-one of which was disqualified, one exited after week 6, one exited after week 8 and one exited after week 9. Three of the final participants were in Group I and the remaining two were in group II

Group I Responses

Three of the participants in this group reintroduced allergen foods with no allergic responses to the previously offending foods. One participant reintroduced allergen food with reduced response to previously offending foods. None of the

70

participants in this group exhibited the same allergic response at the end of the study as prior to the study. The details of these cases are included in Chapter 7.

Group II Responses

This entire group experienced no allergic responses to some previously offending foods, one experienced a significantly reduced allergic response to one previously offending food and one still experienced the same response on one previously offending food. Both had notable results.

Implications of study results

The sample size of this study was too small to make any definitive conclusions regarding the efficacy of this therapy as it would apply to the general population. It is important to note that significant reduction of symptoms of most anaphylactic reactions was achieved. This opens additional questions which could lead to additional or further studies. One could also conclude that food sensitivities may be cured with vitamin and nutrition therapy as the result of this study are reflective of those results produced by previous work as noted in Chapter 1 of this work.

Chapter 6

Conclusion

Reversal success of allergies with vitamin and nutrition therapy

The participants in the clinical study all achieved excellent results in healing. Those that followed the study protocol were able to reintroduce foods that had previously caused an allergic reaction with a lesser reaction or no reaction at all. These results were achieved over a ninety day period in an outpatient setting. These same protocols administered on an in-patient basis would garner the same results in a much shorter time.

An in-patient facility would provide support during the first few weeks of haling, as well as provide an environment in which the patient can focus on care and education that will empower the individual to continue healing once in-patient care has concluded.

This has been proven in facilities in the Southwest US as well as in Mexico.

Dr. Gabriel Cousens runs the Tree of Life Rejuvenation Center in Arizona. The center is a resort type healing center with extended stay accommodations. The center focuses primarily on diabetes reversal in a vitamin and nutrition based program which requires a three week stay at the facility and one year of outpatient after care.

Dr. Max Gerson's work, as discussed in Chapter 4, has been applied to a wide range of diseases and is known for its efficacy with cancers. The Gerson Institute was founded by Dr. Gerson's daughter Charlotte, who will turn 93 in March of 2015. Recently, Charlotte's son took over running the institute which is located in Mexico.

Patients stay at the institute for a minimum of three weeks to begin the therapy and receive outpatient care for up to two years. The Gerson Institute also hosts a symposium each year. At this symposium, patients come back for decades cancer free – not 'I think we got it all', not in 'remission', but caner free. These patients share their recovery stories and struggles at the annual symposium.

Dr. Bernard Jensen also recognized the need to focus solely on healing without distraction from other activities. He set up a sanatorium in California which was nicknamed 'The Ranch'.

The Ranch also provided inpatient stay for a minimum of three weeks to facilitate the hardest part of healing and provide a much needed support system to patients during those weeks. Outpatient after care was provided based on patient need.

Dt. Jensen's death in 2001 at the age of ninety two was a loss of one of the most tireless contributors to natural healing of the 20th century.

My own project, Phoenix House, follow is the footsteps of these great healers. This facility is also an inpatient healing retreat where patients can stay for a minimum of two weeks and receive various natural healing therapies, education and support. Outpatient after care lasts an average of one year based on patient need.

The cost of this kind of care is a fraction of the cost of most medical treatments. The average chemotherapy treatment cost $10,000.00 per month for the drugs alone. A minimum stay at Phoenix House with one year of outpatient after care averages $6000.00.

As of the writing of this book, my team and I are searching for an appropriate location for Phoenix House. Our current goal is to obtain a property and have it operational within two years.

Implications of reversing anaphylactic allergies

My own anaphylactic allergies did not manifest until early adulthood, but, with so many small children being diagnosed with life threatening food allergies, it is presumably an immense strain on both the child and the parents of those children to manage those allergies. It is unimaginable to go through every day as the parent of a young child and be concerned that your child's food might kill him or her. It is even more concerning the impact that this worry would have on the child. The reversal of anaphylactic allergies would improve the quality of life of many children and their parents.

The standard treatment of anaphylactic allergies is currently management as opposed to correction. Allergy sufferers are advised to avoid the offending foods and to be prepared with an emergency dose of epinephrine. The reversal of life threatening allergy responses would allow people to enjoy healthy foods which in the past were not a viable dietary option due to allergy.

Other hypothesis derived from this study.

During my clinical study, reintroduction of anaphylactic producing allergens was achieved with no reaction or lessened reactions to shell fish, tree nuts and dairy, while peanuts still produced violent reaction. Decrease in severity of the reaction indicates that full recovery from such food allergies is possible but requires greater than 90 days to totally eliminate the auto immune response. Peanuts, as a member of the legume family, do not summarily fall into the food categories defined by Dr. Lapore. This begs the question, how does one go about correcting this potentially fatal allergy with vitamin and nutrition therapy. Anaphylactic reactions to foods are linked to enzymatic defect.[43] Enzymes are produced and programmed by the glandular system.[44] Additional research is required to discover the best method of reversing peanut allergies by nutritional support and rebalancing of the glandular system, particularly the hypothalamus. There is however significant support already for this hypothesis. In Diet & Nutrition- a holistic approach, Dr. Ballentine writes; 'it is the clinical impression of some physicians that certain patients with a tendency to exaggerated allergies respond well to manganese supplements…manganese helps to restore balance when histamine, the substance that is released during allergic reactions , is either too high or too low in the blood.'[45]

Anaphylactic reaction to peanuts may be linked to severe enzymatic defect and improper production or conversion of the amino acid histidine into histamine. Food allergies have already been linked to deficiency in the amino acid histidine. (See Table 1-1) If the conversion of histidine to histamine by the enzyme histidine decarboxylase is disrupted or if the enzyme itself is faulty, it may create a severe immune response to a substance consumed which is not a threat to the organism – anaphylactic food allergy.

Newly formed enzymes and amino acids are continually being renewed or replaced. The origination of these factors can, therefore be changed, supported and healed with vitamin and nutritional therapy. Once healing has occurred and he producing glands restored to optimal function. New, undamaged amino acids and enzymes may be produce which do not misread biochemical data and produce immune response.

It is my belief that strictly administered vitamin and nutrition therapy over a longer period of time than allowed in my clinical study would successfully reverse allergies that only showed improvement or where unchanged during the clinical study.

A Word about Knowledge

Knowledge is not power. While knowledge affords us more options and the opportunity to make better choices, the knowledge itself holds no power.

It is common knowledge that eating more nutritious foods and being physically active make us healthier, yet the US is frequently ranked last in health among eleven nations. Obviously the knowledge of how to be healthier is not producing the effect of being healthier. Why? Because most of our population does not <u>apply</u> this knowledge.

It is not the knowledge itself that provides power. It is the application of that knowledge- the act of making better choices based on that knowledge, which unleashes the unstoppable human spirit and taps into the innate healing ability of the body. That is where the power lies, in the choices we make.

I encourage you to take actions and make choices that propel you toward your personal health goals. Your first action might be to clearly what those health goals are. Maybe reading this brought to mind someone that you know and providing that person with a copy of this book is your action. You could begin applying the principals in this book and find a naturopathic doctor to be your coach. Perhaps it is something else, but <u>do something.</u>

I have provided resources in the appendix of this book to help you locate practitioners in your area as well as my contact information.

Happy Healing

Newly formed enzymes and amino are continually being renewed or replaced. The originatio

Chapter 7

Case Studies

The following cases studies are taken from participants of the clinical and from significant cases seen in my clinic.

Fred

A forty year old male presented with allergic reaction to yeast, rice, wheat, fat, oatmeal, corn, citrus, and milk with fat being the most reactive. MRT indicated deficiencies in vitamins B, C, D, E, F, & K as well as iodine, magnesium, manganese, potassium, sodium, and zinc. pH litmus test indicated internal pH was overly acidic. Tongue analysis indicated severe digestive weakness while observation of the finger nails indicated general toxicity and malnutrition was well as poor calcium absorption or depleted stores (most like depleted stores of calcium as this would be consistent with chronic acidosis). Iris analysis indicated weakness in the spleen, kidney and liver as well as the reproductive and sex organ. Moderate toxicity of the intestinal system was indicated by brown throughout the intestinal ring of the iris. Bio-Scan report confirmed manual testing; nutritional support as well as immune stimulation, digestive support, glandular system, reproductive system and nervous system support were indicated.

Participant presented no additional complicating factors. During the study all supplements and meal replacement products were eliminated. And a diet of whole raw fresh fruits and vegetables was implemented along with detoxifying measures was implemented. The detoxifying protocol included the consumption of warm water infused with a fresh slice of cucumber upon rising and the consumption of one of three herbal teas directly following the warm lemon water. Herbal teas were alternated daily. By week 4 all allergies except wheat and fat scored 1 during MRT testing and by week 8 all allergens scored 1. Allergen foods were reintroduced with no reaction at week 10.

Participant also noted more mental clarity beginning in week 3 and additional weight loss throughout the study (a total of 15 pounds during the study).

Sarah

A forty year old female presented with allergic reaction to yeast, rice, and wheat, fat and corn, with wheat being the most reactive. MRT indicated deficiencies in vitamins B, C, E, & F, as well as iron, potassium, sodium, and zinc. pH litmus test indicated internal pH was overly acidic. Tongue analysis indicated weakness in the heart and digestive tract as well as indication of Candida Albicans infection. No observation of the finger nails occurred as patient had artificial nails preventing accuracy of the procedure. Iris analysis indicated severe toxicity of the intestinal tract spreading to other areas of the body including the reproductive organs. Bio-Scan report confirmed findings from manual testing, indicating inherent weakness and support needed in metabolic processes, circulatory, glandular, respiratory and urinary systems.

Participant presented additional complicating factors including Type II diabetes, benign uterine hyperplasia and sleep apnea.

During the study all supplements and meal replacement products were eliminated. And a diet of whole raw fresh fruits and vegetables was implemented along with detoxifying measures was implemented. The detoxifying protocol included the consumption of warm lemon water upon rising and the consumption of one of two herbal teas directly following the warm lemon water and live juices specific to the presenting symptoms. Herbal teas were alternated daily. By week 4 all allergies except fat scored 1 during MRT testing and by week 9 all allergens scored 1. Allergen foods were reintroduced with no reaction at week 11.

Participant also noted more mental clarity and increase energy beginning in week 3. Sleep apnea symptoms diminished significantly by the end of the study. Fasting blood sugar reached clinical norm ranges by week 9 and A1C results dropped from 7.1 before the study to 5.6 after completing the study. Participant also lost approximately 19 pounds during the study.

Andrea

A 45 year old female, presented with allergic reaction to yeast, rice, wheat, fat, oatmeal, corn, citrus, and milk with milk being the most reactive causing severe nausea, and dizziness. MRT indicated deficiencies in vitamins C, D, E, P, & K as well as iodine, iron, manganese, phosphorus, and zinc. pH litmus test indicated internal pH was overly acidic. Tongue analysis indicated weakness in both kidneys as well as a toxic intestinal tract while observation of the finger nails indicated zinc deficiency as well as depleted calcium stores. Iris analysis indicated dehydration, weakness and toxicity in the intestines. Deep closed lesion noted in the right eye at the liver, spleen, kidney and reproductive reflexes as well as the medulla and motor reflex zones indicated ongoing inflammation in those regions which was confirmed by the participant. Open moderate lesion noted in the left eye presented in the neck, reproductive, spleen, lung, anus and thoracic reflexes indicated more recent inflammation and immune response which was again confirmed by the participant. Bio-Scan report confirmed a need for support in the immune, nervous, circulatory, glandular (thyroid) and digestive systems.

Participant presented additional complicating factors including hypothyroidism, IBS, and cholectomy.

During the study all supplements and meal replacement products were eliminated. A diet of whole raw fresh fruits and vegetables was implemented along with detoxifying measures was implemented. The detoxifying protocol included the consumption of warm water infused with a fresh slice of cucumber or peach upon rising and the consumption of one of three herbal teas directly following the warm water. Herbal teas were alternated daily. By week 2 white healing lines were noted in all deep closed lesions noted in the iris. By week 4 all allergies accept citrus, milk and fat scored 1 during MRT testing. Full systemic healing was noted during iris analysis at week 5. By week 8 no toxicity signs could be seen in the intestinal reflexes of either eye and by week 9 all allergens scored 1. Allergen foods were reintroduced with no reaction at week 11 with the exception of dairy which produced only mild symptoms of sluggishness.

Participant also noted more mental clarity and energy beginning in week 3 and additional weight loss throughout the study.

Denise

A 35 year old female, presented with allergic reaction to wheat, fat, corn, peppers, as well as peanuts with peppers and peanuts being the most reactive causing tissue swelling and airway constriction, severe migraine and nausea. MRT indicated deficiencies in vitamins A, B, C, D, E, & F as well as iodine, iron, manganese, phosphorus, sulphur and zinc. pH litmus test indicated internal pH was slightly acidic. Tongue analysis indicated weakness in right kidneys as well as a toxic intestinal tract while observation of the finger nails indicated general toxicity as well as poor absorption of calcium. Iris analysis indicated dehydration, severe weakness and toxicity in the intestines. Deep closed lesion noted in the left eye at the kidney reflexes indicated ongoing inflammation in that region which was confirmed by the participant. Open moderate lesions noted in the right eye presented in the pancreas and liver reflexes indicated more recent inflammation and immune response which were again confirmed by the participant. Bio-Scan report confirmed a need for support in the immune, glandular and digestive systems.

Participant presented additional complicating factors including hypothyroidism, high blood pressure, pre- diabetes, elevated cholesterol with no medication, and cholectomy.

During the study all supplements and meal replacement products were eliminated. A diet of whole raw fresh fruits and vegetables was implemented along with detoxifying measures was implemented. The detoxifying protocol included the consumption of warm water infused with a fresh slice of lemon upon rising and the consumption of one of Nettle tea directly following the warm lemon water.

By week 2 white healing lines were noted in all deep closed lesions in the iris. By week 4 all allergies except peppers scored 1 during MRT testing. The iris lightened in color significantly becoming a deeper, more consistent blue. By week 8 no toxicity signs could be seen in the intestinal reflexes of the left eye with only mild signs in the right eye and by week 10 all allergens scored 1. Allergen foods were reintroduced with no reaction at week 12 with the exception of peanuts, which still produced a violent anaphylactic reaction. The reaction was mitigated successfully with one dropper of Osha root tincture. Airway constriction was reduced within 15 seconds and full recovery with no migraine or other latent side effects was achieved with in twenty minutes.

Participant also noted more mental clarity and energy beginning in week 2 and additional weight loss throughout the study of approximately 10 pounds, and pre- diabetes symptoms disappeared. Updated cholesterol levels were not available at the time of this writing.

Veral

A 43 year old male presented with multiple allergies, the most prominent being lactose intolerance which produced severe abdominal cramping, headache, fatigue and nausea.

Based on the results of MRT, Veral tested positive for yeast, rice and milk allergies and deficiencies in vitamins c, d, e, and p as well as iodine, iron, and sulfur. Nail analysis indicated general mal-absorption of nutrients, particularly calcium as no half-moon was present on any digits. Tongue analysis indicated weakness in liver, kidneys, right lung and spleen. Severe weakness was noted in the stomach reflex of the tongue as well as the iris. This was confirmed by the patient as he had undergone gastric bypass surgery 10 years prior and the procedure had caused the stomach to atrophy. Further indications of weakness noted in the Iris include thyroid weakness, prostate and mid-back inflammation and toxicity which had spread to the medulla region of the brain. Medulla toxicity had begun to manifest as severe headaches which often began after consuming an allergen food. Bio-scan findings confirmed other diagnostic findings; toxin elimination was required systemically, circulatory, glandular, immune and liver support required. Weakness was also indicated in the respiratory, circulatory, and urinary system. pH was severely acidic.

Additional complicating factors include Type II diabetes, glaucoma, high blood pressure, high cholesterol and depression as well as the need for digestive aids to compensate for lack specific digestive enzymes due to gastric bypass surgery.

After one week on the study, allergy response (as measured by MRT) began to lessen and nutrient deficiencies began to reverse. After two weeks, yeast allergy tested negative and vitamin C and sulfur deficiencies we no longer indicated by Kinesiotesting (MRT).

Veral discontinued participation in the study after week two, sighting time constraints and personal preferences for foods which were prohibited during the study as reasons for dropping out of the study.

Rolanda

A 41 year old female, presented with allergic reaction to yeast, wheat, fat, oatmeal, corn, citrus, milk and fish oil, with yeast and citrus being the most reactive causing tissue severe cramping and bloating, itchiness, diarrhea, nausea, shortness of breath, tongue swelling and mental fogginess. MRT indicated deficiencies in vitamins A, B, C, D, E, & F as well as calcium, iodine, iron, manganese, potassium, sodium, sulfur and zinc. pH litmus test indicated internal pH was highly acidic. Tongue analysis indicated kidney and intestinal weakness especially on the right side as well as digestive toxicity. Weakness in the pancreas, stomach and heart we also indicated. Observation of the finger nails indicated depletion of calcium stores. Iris analysis indicated dehydration, toxicity in the intestines spilling over into the liver and nervous system. Toxicity had also reached the medulla reflex indicating significant stress accompanied by headaches. This was confirmed by the participant. Bio-Scan report indicated a need for support of multiple systems most notably the circulatory, immune, nervous and glandular system.

Participant presented additional complicating factors including IBS and fallacemia.

During the study all supplements and meal replacement products were eliminated. A diet of whole raw fresh fruits and vegetables was implemented along with detoxifying measures was implemented. The detoxifying protocol included the consumption of warm water infused with a fresh slice of peach upon rising and the consumption of Nettle tea directly following the warm water. Juice fasting was also implemented for this participant. Due to severe toxicity in the gut, she completed multiple juice fasts during this study.

This case was particularly difficult as chronic allergies had evolved into full blown pathologies, however, progress was significant by week nine all allergens except yeast and oatmeal scored a 1 and the limited allergen foods that were reintroduced produced no allergic response.

Participant also noted more energy beginning in week 3 and additional weight loss throughout the study.

Paige

A 38 year old female, presented with allergic reaction to wheat, corn, yeast, as well as tree nuts, with tree nuts being the most reactive causing tissue swelling and airway constriction, severe migraine and nausea and tunnel vision. MRT indicated deficiencies in vitamins B, C, E, & P as well as iodine, iron, manganese, phosphorus, sulphur, sodium, calcium and zinc. PH litmus test indicated internal pH was severely acidic. Tongue analysis indicated weakness in both kidneys as well as a toxic intestinal tract while observation of the finger nails indicated general toxicity, zinc deficiency and depletion of calcium stores. Iris analysis indicated dehydration, severe weakness and toxicity in the intestines. As well as on-going inflammation in the liver and adrenal fatigue. Bio-Scan report confirmed a need for support in the immune, glandular and digestive systems.

Participant presented additional complicating factors including hypothyroidism, recovery from adrenal shut down 4 years prior.

During treatment, a diet of whole raw fresh fruits and vegetables was implemented along with detoxifying measures. The detoxifying protocol included the use of live juices and a completely raw vegan diet for a period of two weeks. This was followed by the use of yellow dock and comfrey herbal capsules to rebuild iron and calcium stores, a primarily raw vegetarian diet and supplemental live juices to replenish missing nutrients and rebuild necessary nutrient stores.

After the two week detox, Paige noted increased energy and a general feeling of improved overall wellbeing. After 4 months her wheat corn and yeast allergies disappeared. After 7 months reactions to almonds produced less severe migraine headaches and shortness of breath, but failed to produce tissue swelling and airway constriction. Walnuts still produced anaphylactic reaction. Paige is still under care at my clinic.

Paula

A 48 year old female, presented with allergic reaction to yeast, rice, wheat, fat, oatmeal, corn, citrus, and fish oil with corn being the most reactive causing severe auto-toxicity, bloating, mental fogginess, cramping, and alternating constipation and diarrhea. MRT indicated deficiencies in vitamins A, B, C, D, E, and F, P & K as well as calcium, iodine, iron, manganese, magnesium, phosphorus, potassium, sodium and zinc. pH litmus test indicated internal pH was highly acidic. Tongue analysis indicated severe intestinal toxicity and Candida infection. The Candida was confirmed by the patient, she was on medication to control thrush. Observation of the finger nails indicated severe malnutrition and depletion of calcium stores. Iris analysis indicated dehydration, severe and wide spread toxicity throughout out the entire body. Patient's blue eyes had become golden brown after decades of antibiotic and drug treatment for chronic conditions. Bio-Scan report indicated support was required for immune system and nervous system.

Paula presented additional symptoms of insomnia frequent sinus infections, high blood pressure and environmental allergies. Paula's immune system had become so taxed that was beginning to shut down and she had begun to manifest chronic disease.

Paula was placed on a vegan diet of primarily raw foods with live juices to supplement for 30 days. Water intake was increased and nettle, fennel and dandelion teas were added into the diet.

After 30 days a 4 day juice fast was implemented which was well tolerated and she noted feeling much better after the fast. She began sleeping through the night and eliminated the medication for thrush. Within 60 days all nutrients and allergies previously tested scored a 1 when tested with MRT.

After 90 days, Paula had eliminated 2 medications, her high blood pressure was coming into normal ranges and large portions of the iris had returned to their blue color. As of the writing of this book, Paula has eliminated half of her medications and indicated no allergic response to dogs and only a minor allergic response to cats. Paula is still under care at my clinic

Appendix A

Generic Fast Protocol

This is a general outline of the fasting protocol. Specific foods in each case may differ based on individual allergies and biochemical individuality.

Day 1-4
Begin Juice Fast

First thing in the morning:
Rise from bed standing with your feet about hip width apart; raise your arms out to the sides of the body continuing until your palms touch with arms straight above the head.
Breathe deeply in through the nose counting to 5
Exhale slowly counting to 5 and reach for the ceiling stretching the torso.
Slowly lower the arms to the sides

Repeat 5 times

Begin the morning with Green Juice (See Appendix)
Each hour after consume 8 ounces of apple/carrot juice until 30 min prior to bed.
30 min prior to bed consume Nature's Ambien Juice

Repeat morning stretch just before retiring for the evening.

The fast was followed by one day of light foods which increased to heavier meals at the end of that day and a diet which resumed the whole foods approach from other days on the study. See the Sample Daily Menu for a detailed view of daily meals.

Juice Recipes from Juice Fast

These are standard recipes which may have been modified to better suit the needs of the individual participant or allow for substitutions for allergen foods

Green Juice

1 green apple
1 carrot
2 large spinach leaves
2 dandelion or cabbage leaves
1 large kale leaf
½ clove of garlic
Handful of watercress.

Nature's Ambien Juice

1 apple (any color)
1 carrot
3 stalks of celery with tops.

Sample Daily Menu

Day 1

7am – Morning Stretches
- Sit in straight backed chair with feet flat on the floor.
- Breathe deeply in through the nose and out through the mouth 10 times
- Bring the arms out to the sides of the body and slowly up above your head
- Staying seated stretch with the arms reaching for the ceiling. Hold for 10 seconds.
- Slowly bring the arms down to the lap and repeat exercise 5 x.

730am- Wake up Juice
- 1 cup of warm spring water with fresh squeeze of lemon
- 1 cup of nettle tea

7:45 am
- Go for brisk walk for 15 minutes

8:30 am Breakfast Starter
- 1 cup of raspberry. Mix with blackberries if you like.

9:15 AM Breakfast Meal
- 1 cup steal cut oat meal made with almond milk
- 3 or more stalks of celery or one whole bell pepper any color

10:30am Snack
- Handful of baby carrots or raw asparagus with Tbsp. hummus
- Green Juice (see Appendix)

12:00pm Lunch
- 1 cup cooked navy beans with basil
- 1 cup of spinach or raw kale
- ½ Cucumber
- 1 whole bell pepper any color
- Handful of dill herb sprinkled throughout
- Squeeze raw fresh lemon or dash of orange

2:30pm Snack
- Handful of almonds or pistachios
- 4 or more radishes

6:00pm Dinner
- Apple Carrot Juice (see Appendix)
- 4 ounces artichoke pasta with shredded carrots and alfalfa sprouts
- 1 cups miso soup with scallions
- Medium sweet potato baked or raw

8:00pm. Snack
- 1-2 fresh raw peaches

8:30-9:00pm Evening Exercise
Repeat morning stretches here.

Resources and Contact Info

The American Association of Drugless Practitioners (AADP) and American Holistic Medical Association (AHMA) are wonderful resources for finding a Naturopathic Doctor (ND) or other holistic practitioner.

American Association of Drugless Practitioners
www.aadp.net 1.888.764.2237

Academy of Integrated Health and Medicine (AIHM) formerly American Holistic Medical Association (AHMA) www.aihm.org

Dr. Dannielle MacDuff, ND
www.phoenixhouseohio.com
drdanni@phoenixhouseohio.com
Facebook.com/phoenixdrdanni
Twitter - @phoenixdrdanni
LinkedIn – Dannielle MacDuff

Glossary

Ad Liberatim - Latin: meaning as much as desired. The English term, liberally, comes form this.

Anecdotal Evidence – information that is not based on facts or careful study" "reports or observations of usually unscientific observers" "casual observations or indications rather than rigorous or scientific analysis

Empirical Diet – A method of determining food allergies by eliminating all foods and reintroducing individual foods one at a time, usually in two week intervals and observing reactions to the food.

Metabolic Antagonist – A term coined by Dr. Lapore to mean a food which produces an allergic response.

Nutritional Antidote – A term coined by Dr. Lapore referring to nutritional factors which, when brought back into balance eliminate the metabolic antagonist for which the antidote is prescribed.

Nutritional Isolate – Dietary supplements usually in capsule or caplet form made from isolate nutritional factors, often from mineral salts of inorganic origin.

Placebo Effect – Also called the placebo response. A phenomenon in which a placebo, a fake treatment, an inactive substance like sugar, distilled water, or saline solution, can sometimes improve a patient's condition simply because the person has the expectation that it will be helpful.

Tincture – Tinctures are liquid extracts made from herbs that you take orally (by mouth). They are usually extracted in alcohol, but they can also be extracted in vegetable glycerin or apple cider vinegar.

END NOTES

[1] *There is a Cure For Diabetes* Dr. Gabriel Cousens MD pg 181
[2] *The Ultimate Healing System* Dr. Donald Lapore, N.D. pg. 16-17
*this table is a combination of that found in the resource sited and the authors own work based on information in the same resource.
[3] http://www.foodallergy.org/facts-and-stats retrieved 12/16/13
[4] http://www.foodallergy.org/facts-and-stats retrieved 12/16/13
[5] http://www.foodallergy.org/facts-and-stats retrieved 12/16/13

[6] *Food Allergy Among U.S. Children: Trends in Prevalence and Hospitalizations* by Amy M. Branum, M.S.P.H. and Susan L. Lukacs, D.O., M.S.P.H.

[7] *The Chemistry of Man* Dr. Bernard Jensen pg 268
[8] http://www.firsttoserve.com/Newsflashes/Newsflash/The_Connection_Between_Food_Allergies_and_Diabetes/ retrieved 12/26/13
[9] *Diet & Nutrition, A Holistic Approach* Dr. Rudolph Ballentine MD pg 532
[10] http://www.theguardian.com/science/2008/dec/11/diabetes-food-health retrieved 4/13/13
[11] *A Cancer Battle Plan* Anne E. Frahm and David J. Frahm pg 78
[12] *There is a Cure For Diabetes* Dr. Gabriel Cousens pg 57
[13] Genetic Roulette- The Gamble Of Our Lives DVD Jeffrey M Smith
[14] Genetic Roulette- The Gamble Of Our Lives DVD Jeffrey M Smith
[15] Genetic Roulette- The Gamble Of Our Lives DVD Jeffrey M Smith

[16] *Ag Chemical And Crop Nutrient Interactions – Current Update*, Don M. Huber, Emeritus Professor, Purdue University November 12, 2012 retrieved 12/15/13

[17] *The Gerson Therapy* Charlotte Gerson and Morton Walker DPM

pg. 25-26

[18] *The Gerson Therapy* Charlotte Gerson and Morton Walker DPM pg. 21 Table 1-2

[19] *The Gerson Therapy* Charlotte Gerson and Morton Walker DPM pg. 2

[20] *The Gerson Therapy* Charlotte Gerson and Morton Walker DPM pg. 2; *The Chemistry of Man* Dr. Bernard Jenson pg. 268

[21] *The Gerson Therapy* Charlotte Gerson and Morton Walker DPM pg. 392

[22] *The Gerson Therapy* Charlotte Gerson and Morton Walker DPM pg. 138

[23] *The Gerson Therapy* Charlotte Gerson and Morton Walker DPM pg. 13

[24] *The Gerson Therapy – Healing "Incurable" Illness* Vol.1 DVD

[25] http://www.wigmore.org/miracles_wheatgrass.html

[26] http://www.healthbanquet.com/ann-wigmore.html

[27] http://www.healthbanquet.com/ann-wigmore.html

[28] *Naturama Living Textbook* Ann Wigmore, http://www.healthbanquet.com/ann-wigmore.html

[29] *Wheat grass juice in the treatment of active distal ulcerative colitis: A randomized double-blind placebo-controlled trial.* Ben-Ayre E.; Goldin E.; Wengrower D.; Stamper A.; Kohn R.; Berry E. 2002. Scand. J. Gastroenterology, Vol:37.4:444-449(6)

[30] http://www.living-foods.com/articles/wheatgrassbenefits.html, http://www.perfecthealthnow.com/herbs.html

[31] *Healing Children Naturally* Dr. Michael Savage PhD pg. 156

[32] *Healing Children Naturally* Dr. Michael Savage PhD pg. 157-160

[33] *Healing Children Naturally* Dr. Michael Savage PhD pg. 237

[34] *Healing Children Naturally* Dr. Michael Savage PhD pg. 178

[35] *Healing Children Naturally* Dr. Michael Savage PhD pg. 178-180

[36] *The Ultimate Healing System* Dr. Donald Lapore, N.D. pg. 9

[37] *The Chemistry of Man* Dr. Bernard Jensen pg. 367

[38] *The Ultimate Healing System* Dr. Donald Lapore, N.D. pg. 1

[39] *The Ultimate Healing System* Dr. Donald Lapore, N.D. pg. 1

[40] *The Ultimate Healing System* Dr. Donald Lapore, N.D. Chapter 1

[41] *The Ultimate Healing System* Dr. Donald Lapore, N.D. pg. 15

[42] *The D'Adamo Diet* Dr James D'Adamo N.D.

[43] *Diet & Nutrition, A Holistic Approach* Dr. Rudolph Ballentine MD pg 532ff

[44] *Diet & Nutrition, A Holistic Approach* Dr. Rudolph Ballentine MD pg 532ff

[45] *Diet & Nutrition, A Holistic Approach* Dr. Rudolph Ballentine MD pg 242

www.ingramcontent.com/pod-product-compliance
Lightning Source LLC
Chambersburg PA
CBHW030403290526
45785CB00004B/1888